AN EXCELLENT TREATMENT OF HIV/AIDS

I0505311

JEAN BOSCO SAHAHA

AN EXCELLENT TREATMENT OF HIV/AIDS

Copyright © 2020 by
JEAN BOSCO SAHAHA All rights
reserved

CONTENTS

CHAPTER XV: An international journal recognizes an excellent treatment of HIV/AIDS

CHAPTER I

My experience at school

I have seen many people living with HIV (PLWHIV) who died while they were on antiretroviral therapy. I had in my mind an idea of saving human lives. I found that PLWHIV died because they had a low level of immunity or a low level of CD4 count. Therefore, they had opportunistic infections such as pulmonary tuberculosis, meningitis, and cancers, which killed them. I found a product that would increase the level of immunity or level of CD4 count of people living with HIV especially PLWHIV who were poor. After increasing the level of immunity or level of CD4 count of PLWHIV, the risk of opportunistic infections decreased and their deaths decreased, too.

I was born in Burundi in 1969. I have studied the primary and high schools in Burundi where I was a refugee and I was frustrated because I didn't have the same rights as the citizens of Burundi.

My dream was to study medicine in my country, which is Rwanda. In 2001, I began studying at the National University of Rwanda. I started by learning English for one year and in 2002, I started medicine that I completed in 2008. I was focused on my studies and I always had distinction since my first year where I got more than eighty percent. I also wanted to contribute by doing research that is why at the end of my studies of medicine, I did a study showing the efficacy of the cow milk in the increase of CD4 for people living with HIV, which was a first study in the world to show that the cow milk was a new and efficient drug against HIV/AIDS.

On the other hand, if we consider the past history of the human being, we will see that people used to learn by self-education. There were no advanced technologies but people were educated.

If looking an example of my country Rwanda, in ancient time, there were no schools, no books and no technologies like internet. People at that time didn't even know how to write and read. Nevertheless, they had their way of learning. They used experience in life that they encountered to know their nature and it was based on individual efforts.

There was also a tradition in Rwanda of giving orally the knowledge to their children, which helped them to know things from their parents such as drugs used to treat themselves, to name but a few.

Furthermore, Rwandans had a type of school called "ITORERO." It was used to teach, among other things, the skill of fighting by using traditional arms to the population and this made Rwanda a powerful country in central and East Africa.

Nowadays, we are more lucky than our ancestors because we have the chance of getting from other people who are very far, the education that we need. We know to read and write. We can find books teaching us different skills and in reading those books we increase our knowledge. We can write to someone asking explanation about a certain subject and read answers to improve our understanding.

I liked so much to study since I was still young. I used to have good marks in my studies and one of the reasons is that I was a refugee in a neighboring country called Burundi where I was born. This situation frustrated me because I didn't have the right to go to my country, Rwanda, but also I didn't have equal rights as citizens who were Burundians.

One of the solutions in the refugee situation was to study seriously and this allowed me to complete my secondary school. After the liberation of my country and the end of genocide, I studied medicine and I always had distinction because I was focused on my studies.

Leaders of my country Rwanda appointed me to different challenging responsibilities. I was first of all in charge of a challenging department at one of the biggest hospitals in the country, the KANOMBE hospital, and the department was emergency and outpatient one.

I had to treat so many patients about fifty per day on average and I succeeded to fulfill my duties. The question was how to have further studies with a lot of jobs. Above being head of emergency and outpatient department, I was sometimes acting clinical director and this new responsibilities came to complicate things because I didn't know yet the solution to my problem of continuing my studies. After I was sent to coordinate a Rwandan medical team for a peacekeeping mission in Sudan. It was also a challenging mission and the situation was unpredictable because the government of Sudan could kill at any time our people, so studies at that time were not possible but I did my hardest and the mission was a success.

Back to my country, the minister of health of Rwanda appointed me to be a director of the most problematic hospital in the country. After only two months, I solved most of the problems such as to provide electricity to the hospital, begin a new department of radiography, decrease infant and maternal death rates, begin a system of teamwork in the hospital and stop instability of the personnel who used to leave the hospital for other hospitals, by giving them a bonus to motivate them etc....

I started to plan how I could study, after stabilizing the hospital, as a solution to my problem that I always had, of how I could study.

I wanted to study in order to know more, have more income by having one day a better job and its related salary but also because I wanted to contribute in solving problems scientifically. An idea came to me and it was about distance learning as a last solution that I had to my problem.

I have tried so many universities in the United States of America but I couldn't afford their scholarships. One American university finally came to solve my problem. That university accepted to reduce money that I had to pay. It gave me the opportunity of doing a Master-PhD dual program in public health. I had grade A or between 90% and 100% in the majority of my assignments, my PhD thesis included. It would allow me to contribute in solving health problems scientifically.

Furthermore at school, I have always been disciplined and focused on my studies. There is the SANTIAGO THEORY OF COGNITION, which shows the connection between all aspects of life.

"The central insight of the Santiago Theory is the identification of cognition, the process of knowing, with the process of life. Cognition according to Maturana and Varela, is the activity involved in the self-generation and self-perpetuation of living networks. In other words; cognition is the very process of life. The organizing activity of living systems at all levels of life is mental activity. The interactions of a living organism-plants, animal or human with its environment are cognitive interactions. In this new view, cognition involves the entire process of life including perception, emotion and behavior and does not even necessarily require a brain and nervous system. In the Santiago theory, cognition is closely linked to autopoiesis, the self-generation of living networks." (Capra 2002, page 30).

I agree with what is said in the Santiago Theory because living organisms are linked to their environment, which influences them.

I can give examples personally when I was single before October 5, 1996, I used to drink a lot of beer. I could even drink twelve bottles of beer in one day and every day I had to drink at least four bottles of beer. I could even mix several types of alcohol a day. I could start by drinking beer and continue with whisky in a great quantity.

Furthermore, I used to smoke cigarettes and I could even smoke twenty cigarettes a day.

I could not even save money because I spent a lot of money in buying alcohol and cigarettes. I didn't have a house and I could not study in any university. That is why I had to make a decision on getting married to a beloved woman.

I first of all went to a hospital for HIV test and fortunately the results showed that I didn't have HIV. I was determined to decrease the quantity of alcohol taken, which was difficult before getting married. Since I was married, my wife has influenced me and I started to realize that drinking a lot of beer was very bad for my health. She normally used a good approach whereby she talked to me the following day indirectly about what I did wrongly due to a big quantity of alcohol taken.

This changed me and day by day I decreased the quantity of alcohol taken. I started by taking only four bottles of beer a week precisely on Friday and Saturday, and I have reached a point where now I have stopped drinking alcohol.

This approach used by my wife also helped me in stopping to smoke cigarettes from 1996 up to now. It is true that I stopped smoking before getting married but I continued to drink a lot of alcohol and I had a high risk of going back to smoking cigarettes at that time. But with the influence of my wife, I decreased critically the quantity of alcohol taken, which allowed me to continue living without smoking.

I was even able to save some money and in 2001, I bought a house. The same year, I went to the National University of Rwanda where I studied English for one year and medicine for six years.

I remember that when I arrived at the National University, which was in the southern province of Rwanda in BUTARE town, 124Kms far from Kigali where my family lived, I could not imagine how I could live far from my family for many years. As I was committed to have further studies, I decided to stay at the National University of

Rwanda at BUTARE because it was the only university that had the faculty of medicine in Rwanda.

When I started to learn English my friends advised me to study political science after the English course because political science was much easier with fewer time than medicine. They were mentioning an easier faculty to allow me to succeed without any trouble and to go seeing my family frequently.

I had a feeling of studying an important faculty even if it would be difficult. My first choice was medicine because I wanted to save lives. Many friends told me it would not be possible for me to study such a hard faculty, which required a long period of time to be completed, with a family but I was determined to.

I went to meet a friend who was studying medicine and I requested him to give me syllabuses he got in the first year. There were many and big syllabuses; one syllabus could have hundreds of pages to be fully understood and memorized. I remember a syllabus of anatomy that had more than three hundred pages and I took two weeks to read, understand and memorize it. I tried to do some exams they had done and I succeeded them. This success came to encourage and show me it would be possible to study medicine. I continued to read the syllabuses one by one and I did an examination after each syllabus that I succeeded. I took also the second year of medicine and I read all the syllabuses. After the second year, I took a decision to study medicine despite some friends who were advising me to go to an easier faculty. When I started medicine in 2002, I was comfortable as I had started by reading all the syllabuses. I could understand easily what a professor was saying and write each and every detail quickly. I used to explain to my classmates who called me professor. When I had an exam, I could study and have an idea of the predicted question I would be asked. I used to answer those questions before the exam and generally I found the same questions the following day in the exam. I used to answer them very quickly and within only fifteen minutes I had to finish my exam, which had to be normally done in two hours. I used to get good marks and each year I got a hundred percent in at least one exam. Having a hundred percent in an exam was amazing! I had distinction since my first year of medicine up to the last year in the faculty while I had to go to see my family once a week and come back to the campus to study for another exam in few days. Students who were advising me to avoid such a difficult faculty were surprised at my success. I remember some professors who came to teach from Europe for instance the one who taught biochemistry. He was with his wife from Belgium and he could start teaching when opening the door of the classroom and this required me to be alert in order to understand, write and take note of what he was saying from the beginning up to the end of the course. He and his wife had a limited time that is why they could not lose time and after delivering their course, they had to give us an exam before going back to Europe. They were aged and they were around seventies but they were still able to teach their course very well and quickly. I asked him if he taught at the same speed when he was back home. He answered me that he was teaching slowly in Belgium because he had enough time there, which was different when he was in Rwanda where he had a few time as a visiting professor. He told me that Rwandan students were hard working people. Rwandan students succeeded at a higher level when compared to Belgian ones because the latter students had less marks than the former ones while they got the same course in a shorter time. I had to study on regular basis as I knew I would do an exam at the end of the course. I had some stressful time when studying such a big course in a few time including stomachache and a small localized gum swelling. On the day of the exam, I was well prepared and I did the exam very quickly and around fifteen minutes I could finish doing it. There was a colleague who could not have such a chance of doing it because he had studied hardly the day before. He slept very late at 4:00 AM and woke up late around 10:00 AM when the exam was finished, which showed me that the course was tough. Fortunately he told the professor that he was an Adventist and could not do the exam on Saturday and the professor accepted and gave the exam to the academic secretary to be given to him another day not on Saturday. I was waiting for my marks and after some days the academic secretary said that I had got 20 out of 20, in one of the biochemistry exams, which was equivalent to hundred percent. At that day I was very happy and I could not have any stress. The stomachache and the gum swelling disappeared. I went to a canteen and I bought one bottle of beer to congratulate myself because normally I could not drink beer as I had to work very hard to succeed. The following year in what is called doctorate I, which is the third year of general medicine, again after working very hard, I got 20 out of 20 in an exam. I only had it in a one given exam of Immunology in the whole year and the mark was equivalent to one hundred percent. Furthermore, I had amazing performance in practices especially those done in obstetrics, on pregnant women. I could perform successfully my first caesarean section, in less than one hour, which is normally done in one hour by most of experienced doctors.

CHAPTER II

The origin of the solution

It was at school that I started to think about the title of my research, its relevancy and supporting scientific literature, as well as the financial means to realize it. On the title of my research, I started to choose doing a research on a new drug and my wish was to have "efficacy of such a new drug" as title of my planned study. In my mind I had to find at least a product that would be a remedy for a very bad disease of some patients who suffered from it. This was not easy at that time because I had to choose which disease was very bad meaning killing many patients and bringing other people to be in hospital for quite some times. Another big issue to me was to propose the remedy of the disease. First and foremost I had to analyze scientific information I had and checked the statistics out.

What I had in my mind was HIV/AIDS because it was killing many people and others were hospitalized. The prevalence of HIV, the percentage of affected people at that time, which was more than one percent in the general population in Rwanda and it was 3% in 2015. HIV/AIDS was pandemic meaning that it was found in each and every continent of our planet "Earth". Some countries in developing world had a higher prevalence than Rwanda and developed countries. We could notice that rich and poor people both were susceptible to get such a very bad disease especially when not having taken preventive measures. Those measures were based on knowing very well the disease particularly how it affects a human being. Examples of preventive measures for HIV/AIDS are to be faithful to your spouse for those people who are married, abstinence to sexual intercourse especially for people who are single or to use condom when someone fails abstinence. Other examples of measures against HIV/AIDS are to avoid using the same surgical blade for different people, get antiretroviral drugs for HIV when someone is wounded and has been in contact with blood of another person or other people who have HIV for example in a road accident or for a doctor when he or she is performing a surgery or a health worker when he or she is treating a patient. Furthermore a preventive measure against HIV should be taken by getting antiretroviral drugs for HIV when someone, accidentally, has got a sexual intercourse without using condom with a person who is known having HIV called HIV positive or a suspected HIV positive partner whose HIV status is not known. Those are the major measures but others are taking antiretroviral drugs for a pregnant woman, since her pregnancy, to decrease risk of affecting her new born baby and to give the latter specific prophylactic antiretroviral drugs very early just after birth. I had some Great Questions to be answered before knowing what would be my research. Great Questions are those questions we asked to know more about something. They help us to open up our minds.

The physicist Niels Bohr asked, " How can an electron move from A to B and never go in between" (Page 3 of the book WHAT THE BLEEP DO WE KNOW written by WILLIAM ARNTZ, BETSY CHASSE AND MARK VICENTE).

This is an example of a Great Question and it has allowed the physicist Niels Bohr to go in deep about the movement of an electron and know much more about that movement.

When Albert Einstein was a boy, he asked himself "what happens if I'm riding my bicycle at the speed of the light and switch on my bike light will it come on?" He nearly drove himself crazy asking himself that for ten years, but out of that resolute pursuit came the relativity theory. (Page 8 of the book WHAT THE BLEEP DO WE KNOW written by WILLIAM ARNTZ, BETSY CHASE AND MARK VICENTE).

This is another example of how Great Question can bring more knowledge to the one who asks that Great Question and at the end it helps the whole humanity or world.

The following step was to find a product that would be a remedy for HIV positive patients. As a large number of HIV positive patients died at that time, that product would decrease the number of deaths and frequency of their hospitalization.

My first Great Question was: "Why poor people living with HIV don't have an increase of their CD4 while they are on antiretroviral (ARV) treatment?"

My second Great Question was: "How can I help them in increasing their CD4?"

For the first question of why there is no increase of CD4 for poor people living with HIV while they are on treatment of antiretroviral, I found that without enough food containing proteins added to other nutrients, it was not possible to increase their CD4.

For the second Great Question of how I can help them in increasing their CD4, I went through literature to find a product that could help providing them all needed nutrients including proteins and which was available in Rwanda.

The product, which I had in my mind, was cow milk. It was enriched in proteins, necessary for immunity, and available everywhere in Rwanda due to a policy of "one cow per family." The cow milk was affordable, too, for a certain number of people due to that policy. The relevancy of that product was found on internet, which showed me that not only cow milk was rich in proteins but also was a complete nutrient and had several proteins that inhibited HIV. This literature came to support my idea of getting a remedy to HIV positive patients and the proposed title to my research became "efficacy of the cow milk in increasing CD4 for people living with HIV".

Furthermore, I had to tell my research proposal to a professor who was excited about it and encouraged me to work on it and promised me he was ready to be my advisor on it. Another lecturer in the faculty of medicine agreed on the relevancy of my research and he too was ready to be my supervisor on it.

I even went to meet the state minister of health in Rwanda at that time who was a lecturer at the faculty of medicine and he agreed on the relevancy of my research and encouraged me to work on it as it would help to know what could help a lot of human beings in Rwanda and elsewhere in the world.

For this research, I had to find funds for it and one of the ways to find money was to save financial means from my income and even from received money from family members and friends. I had to request some funds from the university I was studying in and the rector of the National University of Rwanda recommended the commission in charge of research to work on my request. After some meetings, the commission concluded that I could not be granted funds because I was not a lecturer in the university according to rules with regard funding from research commission of the National University of Rwanda, then. It was very difficult to me to find another sponsor as I was still a student and I decided to go to a center in charge of prevention and treatment of HIV in Rwanda. That center was very happy to know my research proposal and was willing to finance it but it couldn't because it could not find funds to provide me at that time. I went to USAID or the United States agency for international development, which normally provides aid to citizens of foreign countries in different areas including health, but it could not provide funds for my research. As I was eager to know what would come up from my research aiming at contributing scientifically to a serious problem of a lot of deaths of people living with HIV and allowing me to complete my studies in general medicine, the only remaining solution was to fund myself the research based on my savings. As I had 1,500,000RWF equivalent to US$1,765, I realized that the study was fundable. I went to meet a restaurant manager in the Kigali University Teaching hospital who accepted to supply 1 liter of cow milk per day for 3 months to 26 patients at 500RWF equivalent to US$0.6 a liter. I calculated and found that the total required amount was 500RWF times 26 patients times 90 days, it became 1,170,000RWF equivalent to about US$1,376 amount, which I had. The manager of the restaurant in the hospital promised me to boil the cow milk before being consumed and a nutritionist of the hospital accepted to supervise it. As I had the approval of the University particularly the school of medicine to do my research, automatically the Kigali University Teaching hospital accepted, too and most importantly patients living with HIV were excited to know about my study and welcomed it by signing the consent form.

Not only I had to plan for a consent form to be signed but also I proposed some tests to be done before and after the study especially a CD4 test for seeing if there would be any differences between the study and the control groups at the end of the study. My expectation, which was my hypothesis, was to see an increase of CD4 at the end of the study for patients in the study group who consumed cow milk if compared to those patients living with HIV in the control group who didn't consume cow milk. All participants accepted to be tested for their CD4 count, then, differently to their routine CD4 test and the test was aiming at the study objective. Another expectation at that time was to see a decrease of deaths among people living with HIV in the study group if compared to those in the control group. Those who consumed cow milk would have an increase of CD4, which normally increases immunity of a human being to protect him or her against opportunistic infections: the causes of death for people living with HIV. There would be a decrease of CD4 for those who didn't consume cow milk. I was happy to have answered my question of how I could contribute scientifically to a health problem for human beings by having an idea of a treatment of a bad disease and I was eager to make my dream becoming a reality.

Moreover, I had to buy a second hand Toshiba laptop for 300,000RWF, at that time, equivalent to US$353 and I managed to put in it important software for my study including Word for text writing and SPSS, which stands for Statistical Package for Social Sciences and helped me to compare the study and control groups, to name but a few.

In a hospital in Kigali, the Kigali University Teaching hospital, I decided to start my research on March 14, 2008. Patients living with HIV were excited and very cooperative, especially those who were enrolled in the study. They had already signed the consent form and at that day they gave blood sample for CD4 count before the study. They accepted that I took their photos before and after the study, which would be published according to them as it was even in their consent form. A photo camera was borrowed from a classmate and all photos were put in my laptop. As I was doing my clinical practices of my last year of general medicine in that hospital, I had enough time to do a follow-up of the enrolled patients and make sure those in the study group got one liter of cow milk a day and those in the control group did not. Furthermore, I had to know on daily basis that a particular patient was alive or dead and what I observed many patients in the control group died. On the other hand, those in the study group were recovering and before they left the hospital I had to talk with them and make a counseling that they would continue consuming the cow milk up to the end of the study. All discharged participants accepted and I had to give money equivalent to what quantity of that product was remaining. They gave me their contacts and addresses and I had to talk with them at least once a week and they could even phone me before that time to give me an update especially just telling me they were doing well. None of people living with HIV in the study group came back to be hospitalized during the study time.

On May 14, 2008, I ended the study and those who were discharged came back to the hospital for CD4 count at the end of the study and a photo of each and every alive participant was taken. In the hospital, the same exercise was done whereby all participants were giving a blood sample for CD4 count and a photo of every patient was taken. I noticed that all participants in the study group who had consumed one liter of cow milk per day for three months were alive and many patients in the control group who had not consumed that product were dead. I had to wait for CD4 count results to compare the immunity of the patients in the two groups. When I got the results of CD4 count, I saw that there was a difference between participants in the study group whose CD4 counts were increased if compared to those in the control group with CD4 counts, which were decreased. I had to conclude on the results and the remaining step, which was important too, was to prove the difference between the two groups statistically. By using SPSS software, a difference statistically was there between the study and control groups whereby a clear conclusion was on efficacy of cow milk in increasing CD4 for people living with HIV. It was encouraging and I was happy to prove scientifically that the mentioned product was helping people with HIV to increase their immunity, have less time in the hospital and live longer. It was amazing! I went to meet with the professor who was leading the supervision of my dissertation and I informed him about the results. He was very happy as it was the first time in the world to show that cow milk was scientifically helping people living with HIV to increase exponentially their CD4. We reviewed together the title of the dissertation and finally we came up with the following title: "Efficacy of the cow milk in increasing CD4 for people living with HIV on antiretroviral drugs: case of Kigali University Teaching Hospital (Rwanda)".

After such a title, I went to present it to the second supervisor of the dissertation who was a lecturer in the faculty of medicine and a specialist Doctor in internal medicine particularly in infectious diseases. Before the title, I presented to him the results, too, and he was delighted. He agreed on the title and I told him that I would inform him about all the steps of the dissertation I was working with the Professor who was leading the supervision of my work.

After reaching the first step of my work ,which was the title, other steps of my memoir were acknowledgements. I had to acknowledge my family because it helped me so much, the professor who was the leading supervisor, the doctor who co-supervised my work and colleagues as well as the in charge of nutrition in Kigali University Teaching hospital plus staff in laboratory at that hospital to name but a few.

I particularly thanked my wife who helped me very much during my time of studies and research. She could look after our two children then, a son and a daughter, and find food, clothes and medicines for them. She could make a follow-up to their education at school by sensitizing them to study on regular basis and do their home works on time. I took the decision to go to the university in 2000 while I had already a wife and a handsome son called Sahaha Yvan Bruce. It was not easy because I had to have first of all a one-year English course in the school of modern languages at the University of Rwanda called the National University of Rwanda then while I was married. The school of modern languages was at BUTARE far from my home town Kigali and I had to travel from home to school. I was not discouraged by studying far from my family and I was committed to my studies. I succeeded in my studies due to my commitment starting with the first year of one-year English course. In each and every test, I got distinction and the lecturer appreciated my performance. Sometimes, the lecturer could let me explain different topics of the course to my classmates who understood then after my explanations. Furthermore, my classmates elected me unanimously as their head to represent them and I accepted their choice because everyone needed it and the lecturer was very happy. He congratulated me and I was decided to lead my classmates by making them succeed all and bring them help each other. I accepted the new responsibility of leading my classmates because they showed I was the one to do it but also to test if I would do it easily in combining such a new responsibility with the one of being a father with a family, which was very far. Later on I found it was not easy but I decided not to give up before the end of the year in order to avoid disappointing my classmates and the lecturer. As I succeeded in successive tests in the course I decided to start reading syllabuses of the following year, the first year of medicine called preclinical one, and I found them possible to be studied. I even did some of exams of that first year of medicine done previously that I succeeded. Then after I took the second year of medicine called preclinical two, and I succeeded in the exams previously done after reading them. Therefore, after reading the syllabuses of preclinical two, I realized that I could study medicine after my one-year English course. At the same time I continued reading many books of English and among them I remember at least a title of one book that was "Impossible does not exist" and which came to encourage me to have future studies in medicine. At the end of my one-year English course in the school of modern languages at the National University of Rwanda, I had a grade of Distinction with 77.6%, which was the highest percentage of my class. Each and every classmate succeeded too and I proposed a picnic to a nearest place, in the neighboring country Burundi, called KANYARU to celebrate our successes. My classmates accepted my proposal and the lecturer supported us and we went to KANYARU, where the celebration party of our successes was wonderful, and since then we decided to form a group and meet sometimes to communicate as students who were in 2001-2002 English course.

In 2002, I was fortunate to have a second child who was a girl and my beautiful born daughter was called Sahaha Ornella. She came to make my family more complete and my son could not be a child alone at home as he got a sister then.

I have always been traveling from Kigali, where I was living, to BUTARE 124KMs far south from my home town, and BUTARE was where there was the University I was studying in. I remember that I used to go to the University on Sunday evening and I studied from Monday to Friday, then come back home on Friday evening. Several times we had an exam on Friday and it took me only four days to prepare such an exam, from Monday to Thursday, even if it required more days for its preparation. As I was engaged to both study and be responsible of my family, I had to succeed in my exams and solve any problems in my family during the weekend between Friday and Sunday. My wife managed to be a business woman in order to overcome the needs of our family especially during my absence while I was at the university. Even when doing my research, I have almost been absent at home because I had to work very hard while combining the internship and the study, and my wife supported me by taking care of our children during that time and doing business as well. On one hand, I was encouraged by what she was doing and on the other hand, I had to work hard so that I could complete my studies on time and come back home to ease the job done by my wife. I remember that in holidays, as I used to succeed on first seat, I could find a job for instance of working with the commission in charge of doing a national census. When I got that job of being one of temporary staff who would do the census, I with a number of people had to receive a training of about 2 weeks after which a test was done. I with those who succeeded, were recruited as temporary staff and we had to be deployed to different places. I was deployed in the neighborhood and my neighbors were surprised to see me, a father in a family who went to study to the university, then becoming a staff doing the census. Most of my neighbors were very cooperative and as I was very quick in writing what they were answering for the census, I completed very early my job. I had time to relax for my holidays and when they paid me, I had financial support to my studies' expenses. In those expenses, there were money for syllabuses and photocopying other useful notes given by the lecturer. For example there were big syllabuses of about three hundred pages with 50RWf equivalent to US$0.05 for one page and around 45,000RW equivalent to US$18 to get a copy of the 300-page syllabus. Other expenses were restaurant fees including payment of a special diet when it was needed: it was required about 1,500RWF equivalent to US$1.8 a day and 45,000RWF equivalent to around US$53 a month for restaurant expenses while the received scholarship in cash was 25,000RWF equivalent to around US$29 a month. When I studied a lot while preparing a tough exam, I needed a special diet, which was more expensive and could cost three times a normal meal a day. I could not drink alcohol in normal time but when I got 20/20 meaning 100% in an exam, I had to find money for one bottle of beer to celebrate my excellent result. Other expenses I had when I was a student were on transport from my home town, which is KIGALI to BUTARE, where was the University.

As I had to come back home every Friday and go to school on Sunday, it took me twice a week to travel, which had a cost of 3,000RWF equivalent to US$4 and 12,000RWF equivalent to US$16 a month. Furthermore, I used to live at a place or an accommodation, generally reserved to medical doctors student in a room far from the restaurant. I had to walk for quite some time, cross the main tarmac road before reaching the restaurant, then come back to my room. After this time, I had to go to the classroom and this was done three times a day. This required some comfortable and good shoes that is why I had to buy, at least once a year, some new shoes and some clothes as well as a jacket to cover myself when there was cold. All the mentioned items required me some financial means as well. Another issue was on health because even if I had insurance from the University but it was not paying a hundred percent all the expenses in a hospital or pharmacy and I had to find some money when I was getting sick. I used to budget for other needs such as essentials for my cleanliness on my body and I had to budget for clothes as well as socks, too. Those essentials were soaps and body lotions, toothbrush and toothpaste, expenses on weekly hair cut plus shoe polish and so on and so forth. Transport fees increased when clinical practices began far from the University and those practices were in the fifth year called Doctorate III. In this year, I could do practices of anesthesia-reanimation, radiodiagnostics, dermatology, stomatology and psychiatrics to name a few and I did all those practices in KIGALI while the University was in BUTARE.

CHAPTER III

My experience in a hospital

I did my practices of Anesthesia-reanimation in Kigali University Teaching hospital far from the University campus, which was in BUTARE. Even if my home was in KIGALI but it was not near the place of practices and it required me to get a transport from my home to the Kigali University Teaching hospital.

On one hand, it was good for me and my family because I was then living with my wife and two children and I used to go back home after my practices, spend the whole evening and night with my family. On the other hand, my wife and children were very happy to see me living with them since half a decade back.

I could then look at home works of my children and explain them when they had problems in their works from school. My first born was in primary three and my daughter was in nursery two and my wife several times, a housemaid sometimes, used to take them to school and bring them back home as my children were still in their early childhood especially my daughter. As I was going from and coming back home while still in practices in my home town Kigali, my children improved in their results at school because I could assist them in their works when necessary and sensitize them to study on regular basis. At home then, I brought support to my wife in terms of education of our children in general and in particular for their success at school. I with my family were happy for having been at home for the first time for almost half a year since I began my studies at the University.

However I had to pay for transport from home to the hospital where I used to do my practices and that hospital was Kigali University Teaching hospital. Every morning from Monday to Friday, I had to wake up as much earlier as possible at around 5:00AM to avoid being late. I used to take a shower then and get breakfast finally walk for quite some minutes towards the bus station. The bus took me from the station up to the hospital and I had to pay for it while at the University that cost was not necessary as my room as well as classrooms were near the hospital where I was doing practices. I was always on time and when the morning staff meeting started at 7:00 AM, I could always be there in the staff meeting room. Lecturers and classmates appreciated how I have always been there on time. After the morning staff meeting, it was time for practices in the hospital wards and in consultation rooms as well as in operating rooms. I have always worked very hard and supervisors appreciated my hard working attitude, too.

During break time at 12:00AM, I could have time to get a soda once there were few patients. At 5:00 PM, it was normally time for going back home and sometimes I had to go beyond that time when there were many patients either in consultation or in operating room. I went to the bus station near the hospital and I had to pay for the transport back home.

In anesthesia and reanimation department, I had to work very hard so that I could not cause death of anyone as it was a very sensitive department in the hospital. Patients in that department were those who had to be operated or those who had a serious problem for example patients who have to be resuscitated. For patients who had to be operated, there were many tests to be performed such as blood tests. For example, one blood test aimed at knowing how much hemoglobin the patient had before the operation to avoid an operation of someone who had anemia without being aware of it . By doing such a test, we could know the level of platelets, which help in stopping hemorrhage. Bleeding and coagulation times had to be performed, too, before an operation to give an idea to medical staff on the hemorrhage risks of the patient. Another blood test was on knowing white blood cells so that medical staff were oriented on the status of the patient with regard a probable infection he or she might have. HIV test was done to the patients before operation if his or her HIV status was not known and an explanation of its necessity was provided. For those who were HIV positive, a CD4 count test was performed so that we had an idea of a probable opportunistic infection he or she might have. For patients who had kidney problem, substances secreted by the kidney in the blood such as creatinine and urea had to be tested as well as an ultrasound of the kidney to be performed. For patients who had a liver problem, enzymes in the blood secreted by the mentioned organ had to be tested as well as an ultrasound of the liver to be performed, too. Before an operation in the abdomen, X-ray had to be done and an ultrasound to be performed as well when necessary. Any cranial trauma required a Glasgow coma scale, which evaluates the level of coma and consciousness including how he or she can do movement by his or her limbs, opening of his or her eyes and how he or she can speak. When a patient has a Glasgow coma scale of fifteen out of fifteen that means he or she has the best status of consciousness and he or she is normal. If Glasgow coma scale is less than fifteen out of fifteen then it is pathologic, which means he or she is not normal. Sometimes when the patient can't breathe by his or her own, intubation and assisted oxygenation are required to help him or her, breathing and try saving his or her life. A cranial X-ray is performed to rule out any fractures of cranial bones and CT-Scan may sometimes be performed when there is possibility to see clearer what is pathologic. After doing the pre-operative exams, the operation can be performed with more information of the patient's health status. In the operating room, anesthetist staff are the first to give the required treatment including anesthesia to allow a better operation without many complications particularly on the patient's vital signs. I have never encountered any failure during my practices when I was in the anesthesia-reanimation department and at the end of my work in that department, I succeeded to have 17.50/20 equivalent to

87.50%, which is a high distinction. I was proud of my grading at the end of my practices in anesthesia and reanimation department, a delicate department, and this encouraged me to pursue practices in the following departments.

The following department for my medical practices was dermatology. In this department, I worked very hard too and every and each patient was welcomed and helped accordingly. I could successfully make some diagnosis and determine treatment as well as act appropriately. I diagnosed some skin diseases such as eczema and prescribe treatment that helped patients so much. I could make ablation of some facial abnormal thin tumefaction after a local and skin anesthesia and these interventions were done successfully, too. Patients appreciated what I did for them and I was proud of what I was doing for them. The head of the dermatology department at Kigali University Teaching hospital has appreciated my work, too. She proposed to offer me to study dermatology in France once there was a post graduate opportunity in due time. I thanked her and I told her that I was very interested in treating patients in general including those in the dermatology department. At the end of my practices in the dermatology department, I had 17/20, which is equivalent to 85% and it is a high distinction.

The next department was ophthalmology and the practices were a success, too. I have always been on time and very active during my practices. Some patients from other departments in the hospital such as internal medicine could be transferred to the ophthalmologic exam of their eyes especially those who had diabetes. I knew how to examine their eyes and rule out any pathologies that may stop their vision. Furthermore, I could know how to measure a vision, which is not normal with ophthalmologic equipment. I liked it because it was my first time to do such interesting practices. Many patients got their results on tests of their vision problems and they could immediately get treatment as well. There were patients in need of glasses, especially aged patients, and they could get a prescription of those glasses with specifications according to their vision problems. In the Kigali University Teaching hospital, they could not find those glasses, which were bought in ophthalmologic shops outside the hospital. There were some patients who were getting an appointment to be operated for their serious problems of their eyes such as patients with cataract. Patients with cataract cannot see but after an ophthalmologic surgery they can see properly. At the end of my practices in the ophthalmology department, I could get 17/20 or 85%, which is a high distinction. I was very happy of such a high performance during my practices in the ophthalmology department. This reminded me how I was focused on studying such a course in Doctorate III at the faculty of medicine, the National University of Rwanda. In that course and in its exam, I had 18/20 equivalent to 90%, which is a high distinction. It showed me that where there is a will, there is success.

The following department was stomatology. Practices in this department were very interesting too, because I had to work on teeth and facial tumors. Normally, diseases in the mouth are prevented by hygienic measures through brushing after getting a meal especially during the night. This time is key because it is when people spend a lot of time on bed while bacteria develop easily once they have not brushed. The most important advice should be prevention by brushing after having a meal and such a good practice decreases risks of getting unnecessary oral diseases particularly dental ones. Many patients came to the department of stomatology at the Kigali University Teaching hospital with those diseases and the cause was lack of enough oral hygiene. The treatment was first of all to prescribe an antibiotic when there was infection. The antibiotic was specific to germs found in oral area. When there were signs of inflammation, an anti inflammatory drug was prescribed too. Apart from prescribing those different drugs, advice should be given to the patient in terms of oral hygiene to prevent another similar disease. On the other hand there was a case, of late transfer from a private clinic, which I could never forget. Such a bad case was of a lady who was transferred lately from a private clinic in town and she was in critical condition. She came with a history of a tooth ablation, which was not well done in that clinic. She had a cellulitis at that side where there was ablation of the tooth. That means that she had a swelling of her cheek at that part of her face where she was suffering from. There was perturbation of her vital signs especially her temperature because she had high fever. We took samples for lab test and they came back showing an infection in her blood. Immediately, we gave a large spectrum antibiotic with inflammation and high fever treatment. It took some days while she was hospitalized but unfortunately as it was too late, she died. I had in mind a feeling of sadness and concluded that dental diseases should be treated very early and seriously to avoid such a mentioned tragic event. However many other cases were successfully treated and I remember that it was my first time to perform the first tooth ablation and I did it well. The following days in my practice in the stomatology department were fruitful especially in times of performing tooth ablations, where needed, including complicated ones. Furthermore, I could assist to many surgical interventions during my practice. The surgical interventions were on maxillofacial tumors. Those tumors are normally big and bleed a lot. That is why we have to be careful when operating them and it takes time to complete such interventions. During my practice in stomatology department at Kigali University Teaching hospital, there was one maxillofacial surgeon from Cuba. He came to Rwanda because there was a cooperation between Cuba and Rwanda, which was aiming at sending Cuban doctors including specialists to work with Rwandan doctors. The Cuban maxillofacial surgeon was still young and I used to work with him for each and every intervention. There are normally clothes we wear before going to the operating room. Those clothes are sterile and they were in green color for the surgeons and their assistants in the mentioned hospital operating rooms. Before putting them on, we first put off clothes we came with, then after wearing those green clothes including a cap and mask, after we wash hands. We finally enter in the operating theatre room where we wear a green gown then wash hands again but with a stronger antiseptic like alcohol antiseptic and finally wear sterile gloves. I remember that one day I with the Cuban maxillofacial surgeon had a surgical intervention of a big maxillofacial tumor, which took us a lot of time. Even if we could see that the tumor was facial but we had to pass through the mouth by cutting with a surgical blade the patient gum for a small part to reach it. It took us a lot of time to complete the intervention and fortunately we successfully completed it. Normally, after any interventions clothes worn in the operating room are left in the changing room where personal clothes are put on. But on that day the surgeon forgot it and went out the changing room with clothes from the operating room and I managed to remind it to him near the hospital quarter gate. He was surprised and came back to the changing room where he left green clothes from the theatre operating room and wore his personal clothes. I noticed that such an oversight was due to the surgical intervention, which had taken a lot of time. At the end of my practice in stomatology department at Kigali University Teaching hospital, I was happy to get 16/20, which is equivalent to 80% and again a high distinction. The obtained mark was similar to what I had got in previous practices such as anesthesia-reanimation, dermatology and ophthalmology practices. The only question that I asked myself was: Which medical specialization am I going to study in the future? I could not answer such a question because I liked each and every department. On the other hand, I had got high distinction in all departments I had been working through for my medical practices, up to then.

The next department for my medical practices was radiography and the practices were exactly in radiodiagnostics. In this department, there was a lot of work whereby almost all clinical departments in the hospital sent their patients to radiography for investigation.

Those departments are particularly surgery and internal medicine departments. For the surgery department, a doctor needs a radiographic investigation on a case of patient to whom a fracture is suspected, just as an example. If a patient is seriously traumatized physically on the shoulder level on bones located at the joint of the shoulder and the arm, he or she has pain at that level and can't perform movements as usual. When he or she consults, a doctor needs his or her radiographic investigation, an X-ray. It allows a proper treatment such as a reduction manually when there is a need of it and such manual reduction is only done when there is no fracture. If it is done without a radiographic investigation while there is a fracture, the patient will have his or her fracture worsen. That is why in my radiographic practices at Kigali University Teaching hospital, many cases from the Surgery department were received in a large number. I had to participate in performing such a radiographic investigation and it was a good opportunity to know how it was actually done. One of the most interesting practices was a radiographic film that was done without delay giving a clear view of what the patient was suffering from. Another interesting practice was about how to protect ourselves with lead against X-rays. Furthermore, I had to make a diagnosis of the pathology for any cases, which were sent to the radiographic department at my presence. I could diagnose a fracture or find there wasn't any based on radiographic film. This was a good experience for me in terms of radiographic diagnosis of cases from the surgery department. Other many patients came to the radiographic department from Internal medicine one. They had many health problems that needed radiographic investigation, too, for confirmation of a certain diagnosis. Some people had lung problems and with only a clinical examination, it was not enough to be sure of an exact pathology. For instance, some people had pulmonary tuberculosis and with clinical signs a doctor suspected it. Those signs were asthenia, anorexia, high loss of weight, fever at 39 degree Celsius, cough of more than 3 weeks and night sweats as well as hemoptysis or coughing up of blood for some patients.. However the doctor had to request a chest X-ray, among other investigations, to confirm such a bad disease. On the TB patient x-Ray film, there were many abnormalities such as pulmonary opacification due to a decrease in ratio of gas to soft tissue and cavitations, which are formation of cavities within a lung. All those radiographic signs contributed to determine the diagnosis of tuberculosis that helped the doctor, too, on what he or she had thought of. I was proud to have contributed to many diagnoses through interpretation of X-ray films of patients. Another department that sent many patients to the radiographic department is emergency department. From this department, we could receive many patients who were physically traumatized due to road accidents and those patients had to get an X-ray film to rule out any fractures before having a final treatment. Other patients from the emergency department could need a radiographic investigation once they had arrived at that department with signs of severe pneumonia for instance. Such a patient with severe pneumonia may have dyspnea or difficult breathing, chest pain when coughing, fever, confusion and asthenia among other signs. A doctor would request a patient chest

X-ray to confirm the diagnosis. On a patient who had pneumonia, we could see on his or her chest X-ray infiltrates, which are white spots in the lungs just as example. The doctor could confirm that diagnosis of pneumonia based on the result from the radiographic department. It had actually sent the patient film X-ray that showed that the patient had the mentioned disease. When the diagnosis was confirmed, it comforted the doctor who prescribed to that particular patient an appropriate treatment with confidence. I realized that radiographic department was very helpful in the hospital. I decided to work very hard so that, based on my level of knowledge at that time, I contributed to the diagnosis of the diseases in the radiographic department. My contribution helped to well treat patients and to save more lives. At the end of my practices in the radiographic department, I got 16/20 equivalent to 80%, which was again a high distinction and I was proud of it.

The other department for my medical practices was psychiatry department. That department was interesting because it had many patients who needed a good service delivery. As there has been genocide against Tutsi in Rwanda, and it was in 1994, many Rwandans died. The number of dead people killed during that genocide against Tutsi was mentioned to be about one million (1,000,000). They were killed by authorities at that time including political, military, police authorities and militias called "Interahamwe" who ordered the rest of the Rwandan population to kill the Tutsis, too. It was an ethnic cleansing and the whole million of people were killed in about one hundred days only. The genocide perpetrators used guns, grenades and machetes, just as examples, to kill all those people in a few time. It was horrible. There were survivors who had been traumatized both physically and mentally. Those survivors needed treatment for their physical wounds. They were treated according to the possibility of the health sector to do so. Another issue was about providing mental treatment to the genocide survivors because that treatment required many staff and much time. That is why in my practices of psychiatry, I could see many patients who were mentally traumatized and the majority of them were survivors of genocide. Many patients had depression, which is a mental illness and it has different signs. Depression causes feeling of sadness, loss of interest in activities once enjoyed, anorexia, asthenia, loss of weight or increased weight, which doesn't relate to the diet, trouble in sleeping with loss or too much sleeping, decreased physical activity, slowed speech, which is observed by others, feeling guilty, difficulty in making decisions and possible thoughts of suicide. Treatment for patients with depression is interesting and it is successful within time as it combines psychotherapy and medication. I was proud to see a patient with depression improving due to a good treatment offered to him. At the end of practices in psychiatric department, I got 16/20 equivalent to 80%, another high distinction again.

CHAPTER IV

My experience in public health

Other practices were done in public health and they were interesting, too. Those practices were done at the level of health center where there is primary care. In fact in the health system in Rwanda, the majority of cases are found at the health center level. Only complicated cases among them, are transferred to the district hospitals and more complicated ones from the district hospitals to referral hospitals, which include university teaching hospitals. In the practices done in public health, they were done in a health center in the southern province of Rwanda and there were many cases especially cases of respiratory tract infections, malaria and intestinal worms to name but a few. All those cases were handled based on guidelines of case management at the health center level.

Those cases, which were complicated with a failure in their management, could be transferred to the district hospital level. In the public health practices, not only a follow-up of cases was done but also the cause of those cases was searched. For example for a number of malaria cases, it could be found that people were not using appropriately preventive measures. An example of preventive measure for malaria is the use of insecticide-treated net and many people with malaria could not use such a basic preventive measure. The recommendation was to sensitize the population to use insecticide-treated net and once done cases dropped. In the practices of public health, theories of how to calculate ratios and rates were put into practice. The occurrence of a disease such as malaria in the concerned population within a particular period was calculated and that rate or incidence helped us to know new cases of malaria in that given period. That incidence is a key figure that helped us to quantify how bad was malaria in the population of the concerned health center. It was very easy, with that figure, to make the malaria problem understood by the head of the health center and therefore advise her to work with local authorities for the sensitization of the population on the use of insecticide-treated net. The sensitization was made and cases of malaria started to decrease in that health center. The incidence decreased too, because there was a decrease of new cases of malaria. These practices in public health showed me that prevention was actually better than cure. On one hand, it is good to treat appropriately someone who is already ill so that he or she can have an improved medical status and be cured. The disease causes a lot of problems on the health of the sick individual and can make him or her consult a health provider. That consultation requires financial means and time, which should have been used by the individual to increase his or her production. There is a possibility of being hospitalized for that patient who consults especially when he or she is seriously sick and needs a thorough follow-up. The hospitalization requires more money and time, which should have been used by the individual for his or her personal development. On the other hand, it is better to inform people about what can prevent them from getting a disease. One of good examples on prevention is how people use insecticide-treated net that prevents them from getting malaria and they save money and time for their development. So prevention is key for human health and there are many other examples that demonstrate it. Those examples are the big role of immunization in preventing many diseases for example poliomyelitis and the importance of adequate diet as well as physical exercise in preventing non communicable diseases (NCDs) such as diabetes and so on and so forth. Poliomyelitis is a disease that causes paralysis of muscles and a patient with poliomyelitis could have paralysis of muscles of one leg. It is caused by a virus transmitted from a human to another human by fecal matters. The prevention is key to avoid such a disease and that prevention in the case of poliomyelitis is vaccination given to children. There are mainly two types of vaccines against poliomyelitis. The most given vaccine worldwide, the one given orally which is called Sabin Vaccine, and another one given by injection called Salk Vaccine. Those vaccines are other good examples of prevention, which has made a change in terms of reducing considerably cases of poliomyelitis in the world.

Another example of how prevention makes a difference in improving human health is appropriate diet and physical exercise in NCDs (Non-Communicable Diseases) case.

Those NCDs are diabetes, heart diseases and cancer just as examples. Diabetes is a disease characterized by an elevated blood sugar that causes an elevated quantity of urinating called polyuria and high frequency of urinating called POLLAKIURIA as well as exaggerated need of drinking or polydipsia. Diabetes causes abnormal hunger or polyphagia and loss of weight, too. There are two types of diabetes, type I diabetes whereby patients are depending on insulin during their treatment and type II diabetes with patients who are not only treated by insulin but mainly by oral tablets. Those patients in type II diabetes have obesity or overweight and they are those who should have taken preventive measures, of getting appropriate diet and physical exercise, which are even advised to be taken in their illness to avoid diabetes complications. The appropriate diet is the diet that does not have too much calories with less lipids and glucose but with needed vitamins, minerals and proteins. For example it would be better to consume 5 types of fruits a day and in terms of exact quantity it is about 600g of fruits, and vegetables daily to be healthy. This diet helps to prevent heart diseases like high blood pressure and cancer, too.

In a book "Social determinants approaches to public health: from concept to practice" written by Eric Blas, Johannes Sommarfeld and Anand Sivasankara Kurup, a concept is described and it is on "Food and vegetable promotion and the 5-a-day program in Chile for the prevention of chronic non-communicable diseases: across-sector relationships and public-private partnerships." The concept shows the importance of fruit and vegetable consumption in preventing non-communicable diseases.

"Non-pharmacological measures to prevent CNCDs, such as consuming a healthy diet, exercising regularly and stopping the use of tobacco have been documented by the World Health Organization (WHO) Global Strategy on diet, Physical Activity and Health (WHO, 2004), the WHO Fruit and vegetable Initiative (WHO, 2003), and the joint WHO/FAO expert Consultation on Diet, Nutrition and the Prevention of Chronic Diseases (WHO/FAO, 2003). Increasing individual fruit and vegetable consumption to up to 600g daily would reduce the worldwide burden of ischemic heart disease and ischemic stroke by 31% and 19% respectively." (Page 53).

I have a personal example, which describes the importance of fruit and vegetable consumption to my health. My family lives in town of Kigali and I used to work far from it at about 165Kms. At my workplace, there were no much fruits and vegetables if compared to those found in Kigali, the capital city of Rwanda where my family lives. Normally, I used to go and see my family on Friday during the weekend. As I like so much fruits in general, and banana in particular, I had to buy at least five types of fruits including the banana before going to see my family. Sometimes I found at home in Kigali other fruits and vegetables and my fruit and vegetable consumption was very high at home with my family. I have never had constipation at home in Kigali. On the contrary at my workplace, at the beginning, I didn't consume any fruits and vegetables and I had constipation many times. On the other hand, I had a high blood pressure of about 15/10 while the maximum should be 14/9 according to WHO (World Health Organization). I realized that a possible reason of constipation was lack of fruit and vegetable consumption at my workplace. I started to buy fruits, every time I went from Kigali to MUNINI hospital, which was my workplace. I ate at least five types of fruits twice a day and the problem of constipation was solved. Furthermore, my blood pressure became 14/9, which was the normal maximum blood pressure according to WHO. Now as I have added physical exercise at least during thirty minutes a day three days a week on consuming fruits and vegetables daily, my blood pressure is 123/83, which is normal according to World Health Organization.

At the end of my practices in public health, I had 19/20 equivalent to 95%, which is a high distinction. I was very happy of my score and I had an idea that among fields of specialization for my further study at university, public health would be one of them. Not only I had that feeling of possible study in public health in the future but also I started to think about doing a research that would have an aspect of solving medical and public health issues. That is how I had an idea of contributing to solve a problem of many deaths observed on people living with HIV/AIDS.

CHAPTER V

End of the problem in a hospital

This problem was a medical problem and a public health one because there were many deaths for those patients. For example in 2007 at Kigali University Teaching hospital, 389 patients living with HIV were on Antiretroviral drugs and among them 86 equivalent to 22.10% died in the same year. This percentage was very large while they were on antiretroviral treatment and note that the prevalence of HIV was 3% in the general population of Rwanda in 2007. After having had my contribution towards the solution of that big problem, I had to find two supervisors for my research. One supervisor was from Internal medicine department and he was a medical doctor who studied infectious diseases in his medical specialization. His name is Dr. Manzi Olivier.

When I told him my idea he agreed on the pertinence of my research and accepted to be my supervisor. I told him that I would need another supervisor particularly from public health field and he accepted. I went to meet with a professor in public health who was a lecturer both at the school of public health and the faculty of medicine, here as a public health lecturer. I told him about my research and he was happy about it and accepted to be my supervisor and head of research supervision. His name is Professor Munyanshongore Cyprien. I informed him that I had found another supervisor who would do supervision, too, on behalf of the medical side of the research and he accepted. I remember that the research went well within the Kigali University Teaching hospital. Supervisors, colleagues and participants in the research were enthusiastic on the research and they were very cooperative. At the end of the study, I had to present its results to the panel of three lecturers who were all doctors including the head of internal medicine department at Kigali University Teaching hospital, then. They were interested in the results of the research and each and every one among them requested the book that had all details about my study. In the ceremony of celebrating the presentation that ended my study of general medicine, I with my family had a reception at one of the best restaurants in Kigali, then. It was called "Chez Robert" and many relatives were present and one of the three lecturers in my presentation was there, too. I thanked them all for their support they had given to me during my journey at the university particularly during my research and the lecturer, present, congratulated me and explain that my research was impeccable and would deserve to be for a PhD. Since then I started to think how I would pursue my study up to the level of PhD and even publish my research in an international and scientific journal. Furthermore, I realized that I would even study public health and do my thesis on my research by adding on it the measurement of viral load of participants before and after the study and particularly to confirm that CD4 increase after the research. Another event that happened in the meantime, was an interview, which I had to give to one of journalists of BBC on my study and many people heard about it. The following day, colleagues congratulated me and told me that what they had heard from me was correct and some gave me 80% on my research.

CHAPTER VI

Cow's milk inhibits HIV

The cow milk has several proteins that inhibit HIV. Those proteins are lactoferrin, alpha lactalbumin, beta lactoglobulin, casein, glycolactin, angiogenin-1, lactogenin and lactoperoxidase.

All those proteins are crucial in the inhibition of the mentioned virus. When the virus is inhibited, the immunity of a human being can increase; the opportunistic infections can decrease and his or her life is saved.

I am proud to have saved human lives due to giving people living with HIV cow milk. I remember that many people living with HIV died while they were on antiretroviral drugs. I had to think what was the cause of those deaths while they were on treatment. I thought their immunity was not good to be protected against opportunistic infections and those infections were the cause of their deaths. I started to think what I could do to decrease those deaths. I thought that a product with a lot of proteins may help people living with HIV.

That product would be easy to be consumed, acceptable by the patients and available to allow them to find it when needed. I thought of cow milk, which was available everywhere in Rwanda due to a policy called "One cow per family." This policy aims at giving one cow to every family that is in need of it, in Rwanda.

This helped so much as there are people living with HIV (PLWHIV) who are poor. Those PLWHIV who are eligible to antiretroviral (ARV) drugs, get them free of charge, but their CD4, for their immunity, don't increase. Their ARV drugs, only, are not enough to increase CD4 for people living with HIV. Meanwhile, the cow milk is a complete nutrient and it has several proteins that inhibit the enzymes of HIV. So the cow milk can increase rapidly CD4 for people living with HIV. I remember when I started the faculty of medicine in 2002, at the National University of Rwanda; I was determined to contribute for the advancement of the science in general and the improvement of the human life in particular.

I was focused on my studies and I had more than 80% at the end of the first year. I was thinking in the first year of medicine about a study that I would do at the end of my studies of general medicine. On one hand, I was trying to establish a connection between the lessons that I learned in the faculty of medicine such as physiology, molecular biology and biochemistry to name but a few. On the other hand, I started to save money for a study at the end of my studies of general medicine. The reason of my saving was because I imagined that I could need financial means to conduct a helpful study. When I studied HIV (Human

Immunodeficiency Virus) in the third year of general medicine or "Doctorate I", I knew that there was no cure for HIV, which had no vaccine and was causing a decrease of CD4 for people living with HIV leading to opportunistic infections and AIDS (Acquired Immunodeficiency Syndrome) and it is characterized by progressive destruction of the body's immune system.

I finally knew that HIV was causing so many deaths.

It was estimated by the World Health Organization that as of the end of 2018, people living with HIV were 37.9 million. Among them, 36.2 million were adults and 1.7 million were children under 15 years.

During 2018, 1.7 million people contracted HIV and 770,000 or between 580,000 and 1.1 million died from AIDS-related diseases. Since the beginning of the pandemic up to the end of 2018, AIDS-related diseases have killed 32 million people out of 74.9 million total HIV infections.

In Africa, life expectancy has dropped by decades in many countries solely due to deaths from AIDS.

AIDS was first noticed among intravenous drug users in the 1980s. By the 1990, the syndrome had become a global epidemic. In 2004, 4.9 million contracted HIV, 3.1 million died from AIDS-related diseases and 58% of those with AIDS were women.

When I started my clinical practical training, I saw many patients who had HIV infection and many died in university teaching hospitals.

I had an idea of helping people living with HIV since that time and I started to analyze what was the cause of deaths for those patients living with HIV and I found they had opportunistic diseases like pulmonary tuberculosis, pneumonia, meningitis and so on and so forth due to low CD4 count.

In my fifth year of general medicine or "Doctorate III" I imagined that I could give people living with HIV a product that had proteins to increase their CD4. The reason of imagining a protein is because CD4 as I learned in medicine was a type of protein, a molecule in human blood and a receptor for the HIV that infected it and led to the destruction of CD4.

At that time, the product that came to my mind was the cow milk because it had proteins and was well known in Rwanda. Furthermore, the cow milk was available due to the national policy in Rwanda of "One cow per family."

When I tried to read about the cow milk on internet, I found that it was a complete nutrient with carbohydrates, fats and minerals as well as vitamins.

On PubMed, in the US website of the National Institutes of Health, the US National Library of Medicine and the National Center for Biotechnology Information, I found that the cow milk had inhibitors of HIV such as lactoferrin, alpha lactalbumin, beta lactoglobulin, casein, glycolactin, angiogenin-1, lactogenin and lactoperoxidase.

In 2008 when I was at Kigali University Teaching hospital during my internship, I did a study that showed efficacy of the cow milk in increasing CD4 for people living with HIV. When I arrived at the MUNINI hospital in 2010, we had 3 deaths due to HIV. In 2011, we had 4 deaths due to HIV while 58% of patients on antiretroviral therapy (ART) had less than 500 CD4.

I remembered the study that I did at Kigali University Teaching hospital and I decided to do it with objectives of increasing their CD4 and saving their lives.

The prevalence of HIV was 3% in Rwanda both in 2005 and 2010. It was 0.9% in the NYARUGURU District in 2010 according to the Demographic Health Survey of 2010 (DHS 2010). It became 1,4% in 2011 according to the Health Management Information System of 2011 (HMIS 2011) at the hospital of MUNINI. This hospital is located in the NYARUGURU district, southern province of Rwanda.

Furthermore, there was a major problem of people living with HIV (PLWHIV) especially the poor ones who were many in the NYARUGURU District. They didn't have enough increase of CD4 while they were on antiretroviral therapy (ART).

So the ARV drugs given to the people living with HIV in the NYARUGURU District were not enough to increase their CD4.

CHAPTER VII

Cow's milk composition

The cow milk is a complete nutrient for a human being. The cow milk has water (90%), carbohydrates (4.8-5.2g/100g), proteins (3-4g/100g), fats (3.5-6g/100g), minerals (potassium 138mg/100ml, calcium 125mg/100ml, chlorine 103mg/100ml, phosphorus 96mg/100ml, sodium 50mg/100ml, sulfur 30mg/100ml, magnesium 12mg/100ml, micro minerals [including cobalt, copper, iron 0.1mg/100g, manganese, molybdenum, zinc, selenium, iodine 22mg/l] and vitamins (vitamin A 39μg/100g, vitamin B1 0.05mg/100g, vitamin B12 0.17mg/100g, vitamin C 0.6mg/100g, vitamin D 0.03μg/100g, vitamin E 0.07mg/100g, vitamin PP pellagra preventing factor or nicotinamide 0.16mg/100g, vitamin B5 0.35mg/100g, vitamin B9 3μg/100g and vitamin K1 17μg/dl. The cow milk has 750kilocalories/liter, folic acid 37.7μg/dl and its osmotic concentration is 23mOsm/dl.

On the other hand, the cow milk has a protein called lactoferrin that prevents the transmission of HIV1 by the dendritic cells, which are normally able to keep HIV1 for some days and transmit it to CD4. The lactoferrin inhibits strongly the reverse transcriptase of HIV1, inhibits but not strongly the protease and integrase of HIV1; the lactoferrin is bound to V3 of the gp120, which is one of the proteins of HIV envelop.

Three other proteins of the cow milk alpha lactalbumin, beta lactoglobulin and casein inhibit the protease and the integrase of HIV1 sufficiently but they don't inhibit the reverse transcriptase.

Other two proteins of the cow milk are glycolactin and angiogenin-1 and those proteins inhibit moderately the activity of the reverse transcriptase of HIV1, inhibit strongly the protease and the integrase of HIV1.

In comparison with other proteins of the cow milk, the glycolactin is the strongest inhibitor of the protease and integrase but moderate inhibitor of the reverse transcriptase of HIV1.

Another protein of the cow milk, which is lactogenin, is a strong inhibitor of the integrase and moderate inhibitor of the reverse transcriptase. Lactogenin is a weak inhibitor of the protease of HIV1.

The lactoperoxidase is another protein of the cow milk and it inhibits the activity of the reverse transcriptase of HIV1.

CHAPTER VIII

HIV details

Human Immunodeficiency Virus is a lentivirus, a member of the retrovirus family, that causes Acquired Immunodeficiency Syndrome (AIDS). AIDS is a condition in human in which progressive failure of the immune system allows life-threatening opportunistic infections and cancers to thrive HIV infect vital cells in the human system such as helper T cells specifically CD4+ T cell, macrophages and dendritic cells. HIV infection leads to a low level of CD4+ T cells through three main mechanisms: first, direct viral killing of infected cells; second increased rates of apoptosis or programmed cell death for example in infected cells and third killing of infected CD4+ T cells by CD8 cytotoxic, lymphocytes that recognize infected cells.

When CD4+ T cell numbers decline below a critical level, cell-mediated immunity is lost and the body becomes progressively more susceptible to opportunistic infections.

HIV is a member of the genus lentivirus part of the family of retoviridae. Lentiviruses have many morphologies and biological properties in common. Many species are infected by lentiviruses, which are characteristically responsible for long duration illnesses with a long incubation period.

Lentiviruses are transmitted as single-stranded positive-sense enveloped RNA viruses.

Upon entry into the target cell, the viral RNA genome is converted (reverse transcribed) into double-stranded DNA by a virally encoded, reverse transcriptase that is transported along with the viral genome in the virus particle. The resulting viral DNA is then imported into the cell nucleus and integrated into the cellular DNA by a virally encoded integrase and host co-factors. Once integrated, the virus may become latent allowing the virus and its host cell to avoid detection by the immune system. Alternatively, the virus may be transcribed producing new RNA genomes and viral proteins that are packaged and released from the cell as new virus particles that begin the replication cycle anew.

Two types of HIV have been characterized: HIV-1 and HIV-2.

HIV-1 is the virus that was initially discovered. It is the most virulent, more infective and it is the cause of the majority of HIV infections globally. The lower infectivity of HIV-2 compared to HIV-1 implies that fewer of those exposed to HIV-2 will be infected per exposure. Because of its relatively poor capacity for transmission, HIV-2 is largely confined to West Africa.

CHAPTER IX

CD4 clarification

In molecular biology, CD4 stands for cluster of differentiation. CD4 is a glycoprotein found on the surface of immune cells such as T helper cells, monocytes, macrophages and dendritic cells. CD4 was discovered in the late 1970s and was originally known as lw-3 and T4 before named CD4 in 1984. In humans the CD4 protein is encoded by the CD4 gene.

Like many cell surface receptors/markers, CD4 is a member of the immunoglobulin super family. It has four immunoglobulin domains (D1 to D4) that are exposed on the extracellular surface of the cell. D1 and D3 resemble immunoglobulin variable (IgV) domains, D2 and D4 resemble immunoglobulin constant (IgC) domains.

CD4 is a co-receptor that assists the T cell receptor (TCR) in communicating with an antigen-presenting cells using its intracellular domain.

CD4 amplifies the signal generated by the TCR by recruiting an enzyme the trypsine kinase lck, which is essential for activating many molecular components of the signaling cascade of an activated T cell. CD4 also interacts directly with major histocompatibility complex (MHC) class II molecules on the surface of the antigen-presenting cell using its extracellular domain. MHC are molecules that bind to antigens or foreign molecules and allow their recognition by acquired immune system.

The extracellular domain adopts an immunoglobulin-like beta-sandwich with seven strands in 2 beta sheets, in a Greek key topology.

HIV-1 uses CD4 to gain entry into host T-cells and achieves this by binding to the viral envelope protein known as gp120. The binding of CD4 creates a shift in the conformation of gp120 allowing HIV-1 to bind to a co-receptor expressed on the host cell. These co-receptors are chemokine receptors CCR5 or CXCR4. Following a structural change in another viral protein gp41, HIV inserts a fusion peptide into the host cell that allows the outer membrane of the virus to fuse with the cell membrane.

HIV infection leads to a progressive reduction in the number of T cells expressing CD4.

Medical professionals were referring to the CD4 count to decide when they began treatment during HIV infection.

Normal blood values are usually expressed as the number of cells per micro liter (or cubic millimeter, mm^3) of blood with normal values for CD4 cells being 500-1200 cells/mm^3. A CD4 count measures the number of T cells expressing CD4 while CD4 counts are not a direct HIV test. Example, they do not check the presence of viral DNA or specific antibodies against HIV. CD4 counts are used to assess the immune system of a patient. Patients were often undergoing treatments when the CD4 counts reached a level of 350 cells per micro liter and less than 200 cells per micro liter in a HIV-positive individual was diagnosed as AIDS. Medical professionals also referred to CD4 tests to determine efficacy of treatment.

T cells expressing CD4 stimulate T cells expressing CD8, which produce antibodies and can destroy the infected cells by the virus.

Both T cells expressing CD4 and those expressing CD8 can activate macrophages to destroy pathogens.

CHAPTER X

Cow's milk increases CD4

In 2008, it was my first time to do a study that showed efficacy of the cow milk in increasing CD4 for people living with HIV. The sample size was 52 participants and the objectives were, to determine CD4 of people living with HIV who consumed the cow milk and the length of people's lives. 26 patients chosen randomly have received 1 liter of cow milk per day for 3 months while 26 patients of the second group didn't consume that cow milk.

There was a significant association statistically between consuming cow milk and rapid increase of CD4 with a threshold $\alpha=0.05$; P=0.038.

Furthermore a significant association statistically, between consuming cow milk and the length of life was observed with α=0.05; P=0.00

I recommended the consumption of 1 liter of cow milk per day for people living with HIV in internal medicine and surgery departments of Kigali University Teaching hospital where I did the study to increase their CD4 quickly. Another recommendation was to do another study on efficacy of cow milk in increasing CD4 for people living with HIV that would include the variation of their viral load.

The study at Kigali University Teaching hospital, started on March 14, 2008 and ended on June 14, 2008.

Two groups were formed such as:

1) Indigent people living with HIV treated with ART since 6 months at least, and having a maximum of CD4 between 350CD4 and 499CD4/mm^3. They were admitted in internal medicine or surgery departments in the Kigali University Teaching hospital. All those patients in group one received 1 liter of cow milk for three months.

2) Indigent people living with HIV treated with ART at least, and having a maximum of CD4 between 350CD4 and 499CD4/mm^3, too. They were hospitalized in internal medicine or surgery departments in the Kigali University Teaching hospital and all those people living with HIV didn't receive 1 liter of cow milk for three months.

The sample size of 52 was chosen based on the formula $n=t^2.p.q/d^2$ with n, the size, and t, the reduced deviation of 1.96 (risk on an error of 5%) as well as p the prevalence, which was 3% or 0.03. As q is 1-p then q became 1-0.03=0.97 and d the absolute accuracy of 5%=0.05.

I had to add 15% of n for lost to follow up and the final n became 52 and in details n was $1.96^2 \times 0.03 \times 0.97/0.05^2 = 45$ and 15% of n became $45 \times 15/100 = 6.75$ and it was considered as 7 because it was far above 6.

Final n was $45 + 7 = 52$.

On materials, the computer was used to collect and analyze data and the EPIDATA as well as the SPSS version 11.05 were the utilized software. MICROSOFT WORD XP was used too for writing the text. The chi-square test was used for establishing a statistical significance on the difference between 2 groups when P value was below 0.05.

A digital camera was used to get pictures of patients before and after the study and the FACSCOUNT machine measured CD4 on a sample of 50μl of blood.

A questionnaire was utilized to collect socio-demographic and clinical data.

On socio-demographic characteristics, the results in the study group were seventy-three percent between twenty and forty years. Twenty-three percent beyond forty years and one participant had less than twenty years. The average age in the study group was about thirty-three with eighteen and fifty-seven as extreme ages, the youngest and the oldest respectively.

Fifty-four percent of participants in the study group were female while forty-four were male.

Thirty-one percent of the participants in the study group have been to the primary school without completing it, while thirty-one percent had the primary school level. Fifteen percent have never been to school and other fifteen percent have been to secondary school without completing it. One participant in the study group has been to the college and another one had a degree.

Seventy-seven percent of people didn't have any jobs and twenty-three percent were working in a sector that was not formal.

Thirty-eight percent of participants were married, thirty-five percent were single and nineteen percent were widow while eight percent were divorced.

Sixty-five percent were living in NYARUGENGE district, twenty-three percent lived out of Kigali and eight percent in KICUKIRO district while one participant was living in GASABO district.

In the control group, sixty-nine percent of participants were aged between twenty and forty. Twenty-seven percent were above forty years while one participant was below twenty. The mean of the age was about thirty-three years with the youngest about nineteen and the oldest fifty-one.

Sixty-two percent were female and thirty-eight percent were male.

Thirty-five percent have completed primary school, twenty-seven percent have never been to school and other twenty-seven percent have been to school without completing the primary school. Eight percent have been to secondary school without completing it while one participant has completed the high school.

Seventy-seven percent didn't have any jobs and twenty-three percent were working in a sector that was not formal.

Fifty-eight percent were single and twenty-seven percent married while fifteen percent were widows.

Thirty-eight percent were living in the NYARUGENGE district, twenty-three percent were living out of Kigali and nineteen percent in KICUKIRO district. Other nineteen percent were living in GASABO district.

In terms of results on CD4 at the end of the study, among twenty-six participants in the study group, twelve equivalent to forty-six percent had among two hundred and three hundred and forty-nine CD4, seven participants equivalent to twenty-seven percent had less than two hundred CD4 and the remaining seven participants equivalent to twenty-seven percent had between three hundred and fifty and four hundred and ninety nine CD4.

In the control group, at the end of the study, among twenty-six patients only seven were alive. Among seven participants who were alive, four of them had less than two hundred CD4 and three had between three hundred and fifty and four hundred and ninety-nine CD4.

P value was statistically significant because it was 0.038, which showed there was a difference between the study and the control groups.

Then there was an efficacy of cow milk in increasing CD4 for people living with HIV.

On the other hand, all twenty-six patients in the study group were alive at the end of the study while in the control group nineteen died and only seven participants were alive.

P value was 0.00, which was very significant statistically.

This means that those participants who consumed cow milk had a rapid increase of CD4 and less opportunistic infections and no deaths if compared to those who didn't consume the cow milk, they got a lot opportunistic infections and more deaths.

CHAPTER XI

My experience in rural area

In 2010, when I arrived at the MUNINI hospital in the district of NYARUGURU, the southern province of Rwanda, I found many deaths of people living with HIV.

I remembered the study I did in Kigali University Teaching hospital and I had to make a decision of doing another study on efficacy of the cow milk for people living with HIV aiming at decreasing their deaths.

My goal at that time was based on ARV drugs that are not enough to increase CD4 for people living with HIV but with the cow milk, which inhibits enzymes of HIV and is a complete nutrient, can quickly increase CD4 for people living with HIV.

The hypothesis was mainly on how the cow milk increases CD4 of people living with HIV and the cow milk decreases viral load of people living with HIV.

The objectives were mainly:

To determine CD4 count of people living with HIV who consumed the cow milk and

To determine viral load of people living with HIV who consumed the cow milk.

In the methodology, the study type was evaluative of an intervention, which means that there was an evaluation of an intervention. It was about giving the cow milk to people living with HIV. This intervention had an impact to those PLWHIV especially in increasing their CD4.

The study design was a randomized controlled trial.

"A randomized controlled trial (RCT), (or randomized comparative trial) is a specific type of scientific experiment and the gold standard for a clinical trial. RCT are often used to test the efficacy of various types of intervention within a patient population. RCT may also provide an opportunity to gather useful information about adverse effects, such as drug reactions."

The sample design was simple random sampling.

"In a simple random sample (SRS) of a given size, all such subjects of the frame are given an equal probability. Each element of the frame thus has an equal probability of selection. The frame is not subdivided or partitioned. Furthermore any given pair of elements has the same chance of selection as any other pair (and similarly for triples and so on). This minimizes bias and simplifies analysis of results. In particular the variance between individual results within the sample is a good indicator of variance in the overall population which makes it relatively easy to estimate the accuracy of results."

The study started on August 09, 2012 and ended on November 14, 2012.

The formula used was:

$n=t^2.p.q/d^2$

n=size of the sample

t=reduced deviation: 1.96/risk of error of 5%

p=prevalence

q=1-p

d=absolute accuracy

I worked on people living with HIV in the NYARUGURU district and in 2012, the prevalence used was the prevalence of HIV in 2011. The prevalence of HIV used was 1.4% in 2011 according to the health management information system at the district hospital of MUNINI in the NYARUGURU district.

With p=1.4% so p=0.014

q=1-p, q becomes 1-0.014=0.986

t=1.96, then t^2 is 1.96x1.96=3.8416

d=5%=0.05 and d^2=0.05x0.05=0.0025

$n=t^2.p.q/d^2$

t^2=3.8416

p=0.014

q=0.986

d^2=0.0025

n=3.8416x0.014x0.986/0.0025

n=21.211779

I added 15% of n for lost to follow-up to avoid having a small number of participants if one of them fails to continue to be in the study.

15% of n=21.211779x15/100=3.1817668.

Finally n=21.211779+3.1817668=24.393546,

n=24.

In methodology, I based on a randomized controlled trial and simple random sample design; and among a group of 24 people living with HIV with similar socio-economic and clinical characteristics, two groups of 12 people living with HIV each, were randomly allocated, one to receive the cow milk as a study group and the other group not to receive the cow milk as a control group.

In the study group, there were 12 adults living with HIV, indigents treated with HIV since at least 6 months with CD4 count below $500/mm^3$. All were living in the NYARUGURU district in Rwanda and were consulting the ART department at the MUNINI hospital. They didn't have any allergy and/or intolerance on the cow milk and they accepted to consume it.

In the questionnaire, a question about the number of members of his or her family had to be answered, which allowed us to know the quantity of cow milk to allocate to each participant. Normally, each participant in the study group had to get one liter per day for three months.

We found a place nearby the hospital of MUNINI at a nurse's home whereby cow milk was boiled at some participants in the study group who accepted to consume one liter of cow milk in front of a nurse who was in charge of purchasing the cow milk, boiling and giving it to the participants daily.

On the other hand, other participants refused to come to drink the cow milk at the nurse's home. We managed to buy cow milk for those who refused to come to drink the cow milk at the nurse's home. We bought for those who refused to consume it at the nurse's home, more than one liter a day based on the number of his or her family members. For example for a participant who had two children, we bought for him or her three liters a day; one liter of cow milk for him or her and two more liters for his or her children.

Furthermore, we had two more supervisors from the MUNINI hospital: one was a nurse working in ART department and the other one was a nutritionist. There was another person from the community who was in charge of transporting the cow milk from the nurse's home to the participants who chose to consume the cow milk at their homes. We had to ask all participants if they trusted that person and all participants in the study group agreed on the person who was in charge of transporting the cow milk from the nurse's home to where they lived. Every day the person in charge of transport had to make sure that all patients in the study group received the cow milk to be consumed the same day.

Once a week, the supervisors from the hospital had to go with a vehicle from the hospital to people's homes and they had to check if no participant had been lost to follow up. The supervisors from the hospital had to sensitize and to make sure that people living with HIV in the study group were understanding the importance of consuming the cow milk. They also had to ask participants about their problems. They had to report all those problems to the hospital where I had to solve them. For example, as it was in a period they were cultivating, they had a problem of leaving their field and coming back home to drink the cow milk. I decided to tell the supervisors to go to see them and send the cow milk to them early in the morning before the time for them to go to cultivate. After changing the supervision time, the supervisors told me that the problem was solved.

Before the beginning of the study, apart from explaining them about it, a consent form was signed and a questionnaire filled, CD4 count and viral load of people living with HIV in the study group were measured.

In the control group, there were 12 adults living with HIV, indigents treated with ART since at least 6 months with CD4 count below 500mm^3. All were living in the NYARUGURU district in Rwanda and like participants in the study group, they were consulting the ART department at the MUNINI hospital. Some of them had allergy and/or intolerance on the cow milk and others told us that they didn't like to drink it; finally others could drink it but they could not afford to buy one liter a day for three months because of poverty. One liter of the cow milk had a price of about $0.58. Participants were indigents and they could not afford to pay themselves such amount of money. They had to answer to the same questionnaire used for the study group for example, we could use the questionnaire then know and record their names, age sex, level of education, profession, marital status, monthly income and number of members of his or her family as well as allergy and/or intolerance on the cow milk to name but a few. They had to sign a consent form, confirming that they were

73

participating to the study and explanations were given to them that we would not buy for them the cow milk but a follow-up had to be done by supervisors for their health; before the beginning of the study not only questionnaire was filled and consent form signed, but also their CD4; viral load were measured.

On materials, the computer was used to analyze data. I used Microsoft Word XP software to write text and even in writing all the results such as CD4 count and viral load. When I went to see a colleague with whom I was in medicine, he was working in a private clinic and he was the one who had helped me to do a statistical analysis of the results in 2008, using SPSS (Statistical Package for the Social Science), at the end of my studies of medicine; he told me that he could try to use SPSS. I asked him when he could be available; he gave me a date and time of our meeting. Coming from another meeting before it ended, in order to respect time, I went to a place called Kigali city tower and I called him. When he arrived he asked me if I had SPSS software in my laptop, I told him that I had it. He told me that he was not remembering very well how to use SPSS and he promised to try to use it. I promised him to buy tea or whatever he could need for the meeting as recognition of his help. As we were opening the SPSS software, someone called me and told me to come back to the meeting place where an American NGO (Non Governmental Organization) called FHI (Family Health International) was explaining its end of activities in Rwanda. He told me they were giving per diem to the participants. I explained it to the doctor who was helping me in using SPSS and promised him that I would come back very soon. He accepted and I went to get my per diem, which was about $174. When I came back to see my colleague who was using the SPSS, he told me that he was not able to use it and he mentioned on the other hand that the study was meaningful. He advised me to contact another colleague who had studied clinical research in the USA with a broad knowledge in statistics. I paid what we consumed as tea and it was about $8 but also I gave him about $16 as transport fee and his time spent with me trying to use the SPSS software. I phoned the other colleague who told me that I could put all data in Excel software. The following day after putting all data in Excel, I went to see him and he told me that it was good for the study to use a software called Stata/1C-11.0, the one that he had in his laptop for the statistical analysis. After statistically analyzing the results especially on CD4, the doctor told me that there was a significant association statistically on CD4 results because P was inferior to 0.05. I gave him about $80 to thank him for his support given to me.

"When whole blood is added to the reagents, fluorochrome-labeled antibodies in the reagents bind specifically to lymphocyte surface antigens. After a fixative solution is added to the reagent tubes, the sample is run on the instrument. Here, the cells come in contact with the laser light, which causes the fluorochrome-labeled cells to fluoresce. This fluorescent light provides the information necessary for the instrument to count the cells. In addition to containing the antibody reagent, the reagent tubes also contain a known number of fluorochrome-integrated reference beads. These beads function as a fluorescence standard for locating the lymphocytes and also as a quantitation standard for enumerating the cells. Analysis is automatic. The software identifies T-lymphocytes population and calculates the absolute counts. Results printed immediately after samples are run and include absolute cell counts for: -CD4 (helper/inducer T lymphocytes)...On BD Facscount electronic pipette. The pipette is preprogrammed to accurately deliver 50µl of fluid..."

The viral load was measured by TAQMAN system. This viral load measurement was not done in our hospital of MUNINI and we had to send samples to the National Reference Laboratory in the capital city of Rwanda: Kigali. Even in this laboratory, the challenge was to measure viral load below 20 copies of RNA of HIV/ml of blood and it was undetectable.

On the other hand, I had to negotiate with the National Reference Laboratory in order to have results in due time without delaying and they accepted.

"In early 2008, Suisse researchers issued a statement that a person taking HIV treatment who had an undetectable viral load (below 40 copies/ml) for at least six months, who took all doses of their HIV treatment and did not have a STI, should be considered unable to transmit HIV sexually."

According to COBAS, TAQMAN user guide, a methodology, a thermal cycler system and a fluorometer system were described:

Methodology

"The COBAS TAQMAN analyzer uses Roche's patented technology which employs the use of the 5 nuclease assay PCR; The method uses a dual fluorescent dye-labeled probe that contains a reporter dye and a quencher dye. The fluorescence of the probe is quenched when it is in its native state. During the reaction, exonuclease activity of DNA polymerase cleaves the probe and separates the two dyes. This eliminates the quenching of the reporter dye and results increase in fluorescent signal."

Thermal cycler system: "The thermal cycler system serves to cycle the temperature of the prepared samples and to read the sample fluorescence. The thermal cycler system contains for thermal cycler segments...Each thermal cycler segment can hold up to 24k-tubes containing processed sample and master mix, allowing for simultaneous amplification and defection of up to 96 ample k-carriers are loaded and unloaded automatically by the transfer head. The heated cover of thermal cycler segment is thermally connected to the carrier and opens and closes automatically."

Fluorometer system: " Four 24-channel fluorometers read all k-tubes simultaneously using four different filter combination. The excitation source is a tungsten-halogen lamp. The reference channel monitors excitation light source and reference values are used in the result calculation to correct for any excitation drift. To protect the samples from photolysis during the non-reading time, a shutter blocks the excitation light. The excitation filter wheel holds four filters and is rotated by a stopper motor.

The emission (filter wheel) wavelength of the fluorophore is selected by a second optical filter. The emission filter wheel holds four filters and is also rotated by a stepper motor. The photo detector is an application specific integrated circuit (PhotoAsic). The PhotoAsic consists of an array of 6x6 Silicon photo diodes. An integrated multiplexer allows the readout of every single signal of the photo diodes."

At the beginning of the study, I had results of viral load for participants at a possible minimum time of two weeks and at the end of the study, it delayed and took one month and one week.

A Questionnaire was used to collect data of socio-demographic and clinical characteristics.

In overall outcomes, there was a link of the study and the real life and scientifically the impact in general was to determine the efficacy of the cow milk in the increase of CD4 for people living with HIV. In terms of medical impact, on one hand, it was on knowing how much quantity of the cow milk to be consumed per day and on the other hand, how much time the cow milk has to be consumed for a rapid increase of CD4 for people living with HIV.

As results on socio-demographic characteristics, in the NYARUGURU district, at the MUNINI hospital and in the study group; eighty-three percent of all participants were between thirty and fifty years of age. Eight percent of all participants in the study group had more than fifty years. The average age for the study group was about forty one years and twenty-eight years as the age of the youngest participant and fifty-seven years as the age of the oldest participant. Fifty-eight percent of all participants in the study group were female and forty-two percent were male.

Forty-two percent of all participants in the study group had completed the primary school and forty-two percent had never been to school. Two participants in the study group had been to school without completing the primary school.

All participants in the study group were farmers and sixty-seven percent of them were married while seventeen percent were divorced. One participant in the study group was single while another one was a widow.

All participants in the study group were living in the NYARUGURU district.

In the control group, twenty-five percent of all participants had between thirty and fifty years. Seventeen percent in the control group had more than fifty years. One participant in the control group had less than thirty years. The average age for the control group was forty-two years and the youngest participant in the control group had twenty-four years while the oldest participant was sixty years old.

Fifty-eight percent in the control group were female and forty-two percent were male. Forty-two percent in the control group had never been to school and thirty percent had completed the primary school while twenty-five percent of all participants in the control group had been to school without completing it.

All participants in the control group were farmers and sixty-seven percent were married while five percent of all participants in the control group had been to school without completing it.

Seventeen percent of participants in the control group were divorced, one participant was single while another one was a widow.

All participants in the control group were living in the NYARUGURU District.

Table1. Socio-Demographic characteristics of the study population

Table1.1 Distribution of the study population based on Age

Age (in years)	Study group (Frequency)	Study group (Percentage)	Control group (Frequency)	Control group (Percentage)	Total (Frequency)
<30	1	8.3	1	8.3	2
30-50	10	83.3	9	75	19
>50	1	8.3	2	16.6	3
Total	12	100	12	100	24

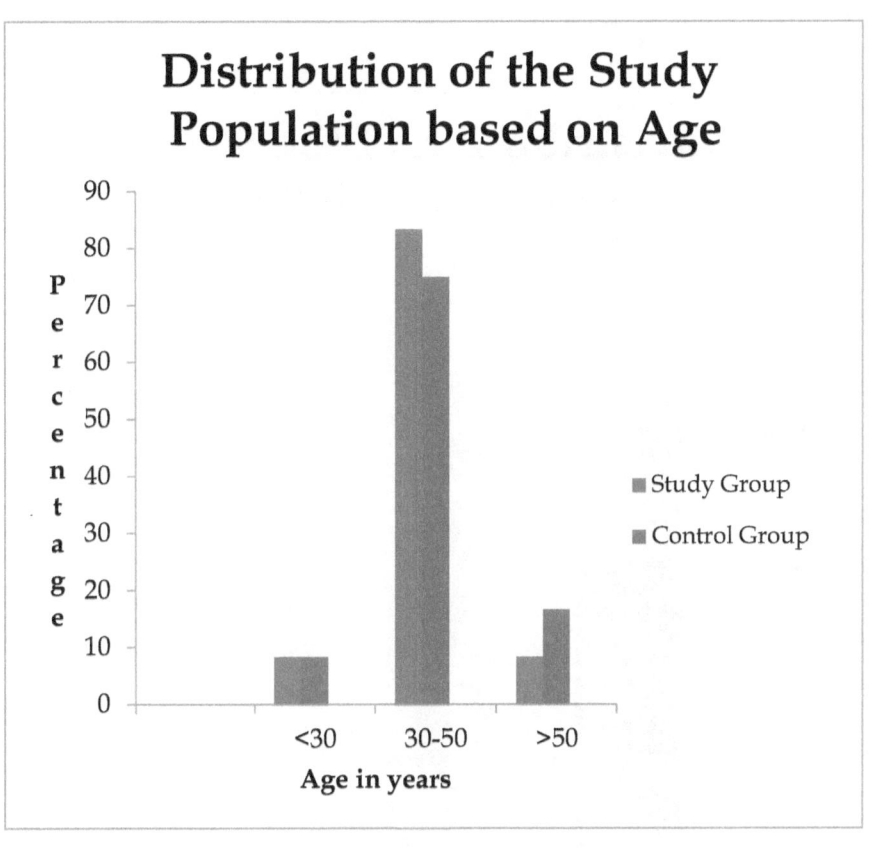

Table 1.2 Distribution of the study population based on sex

Sex	Study group (Frequency)	Study group (Percentage)	Control group (Frequency)	Study group (Percentage)	Total (Frequency)
Female	7	58.3	7	58.3	14
Male	5	41.6	5	41.6	10
Total	12	100	12	100	24

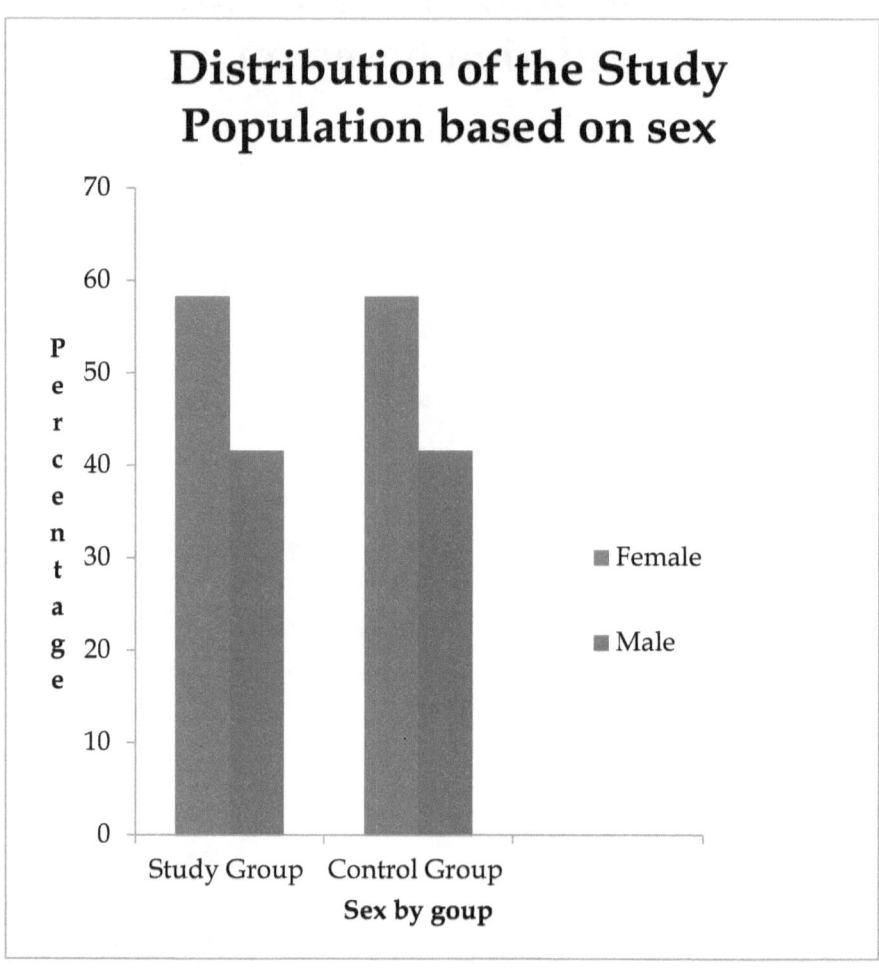

Table 1.3 Distribution of the study population based on the level of education

Level of education	Study group (Frequency)	Study group (Percentage)	Control group (Frequency)	Control group (Percentage)	Total (Frequency)
Never to school	5	41.7	5	41.7	10
Primary not completed	2	16.7	3	25	5
Primary completed	5	41.7	4	33	9
Total	12	100	12	100	24

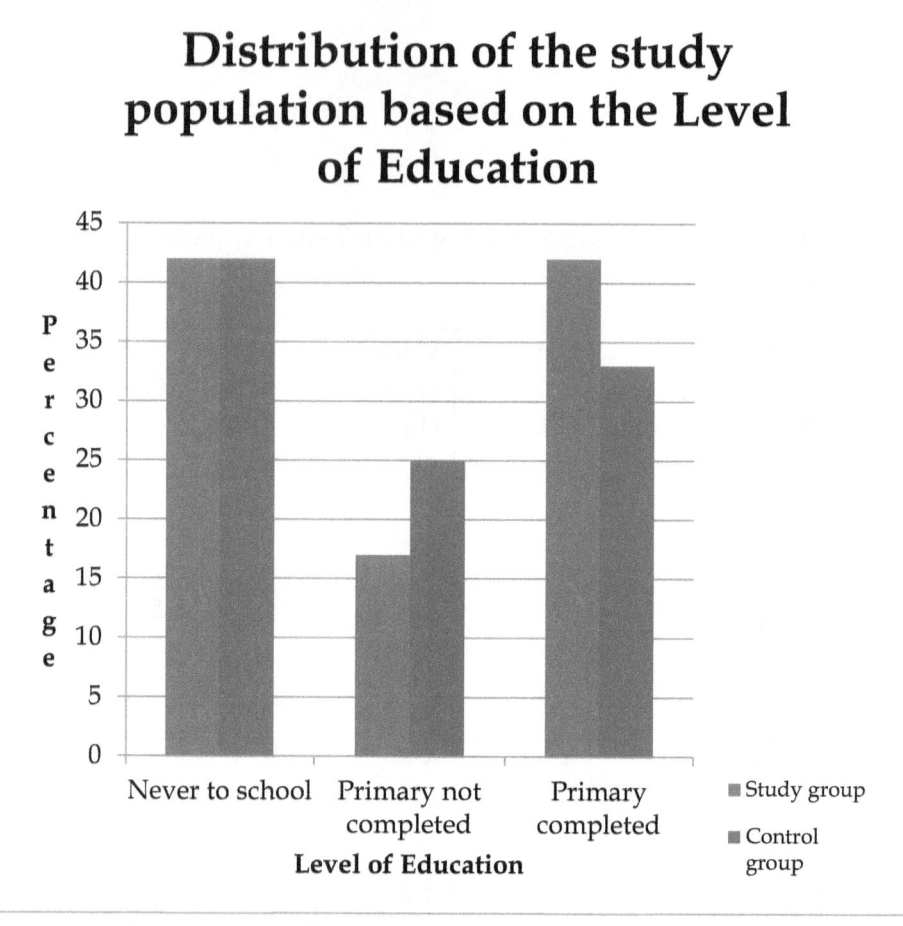

Table 1.4 Distribution of the study population based on the profession

Profession	Study group (Frequency)	Study group (Percentage)	Control group (Frequency)	Control group (Percentage)	Total (Frequency)
Farmers	12	100	12	100	24
Total	12	100	12	100	24

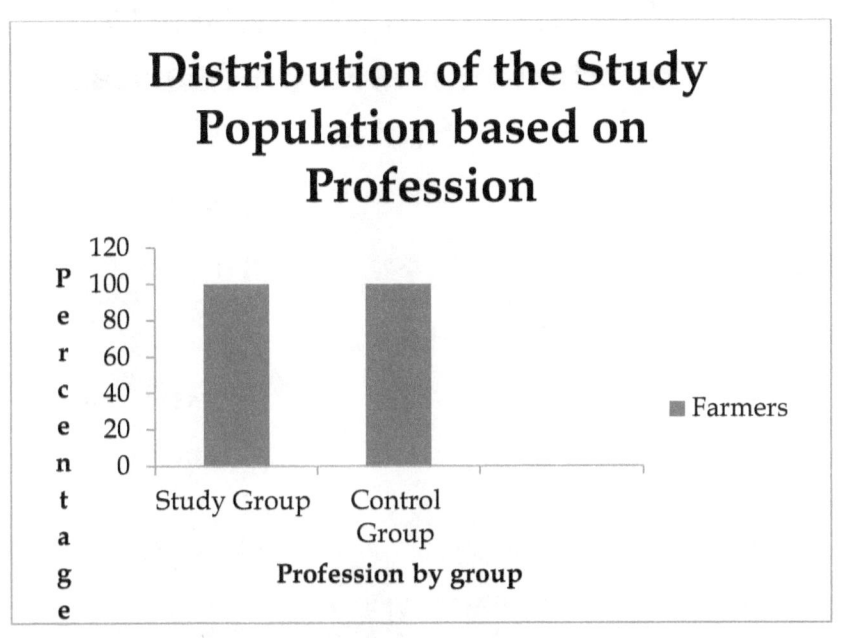

Table 1.5 Distribution of the study population based on marital status

Marital status	Study group (Frequency)	Study group (Percentage)	Control group (Frequency)	Control group (Percentage)	Total (Frequency)
Single	1	8.3	1	8.3	2
Married	8	66.6	8	66.6	16
Divorced	2	16.6	2	16.6	4
Widow	1	8.3	1	8.3	2
Total	12	100	12	100	24

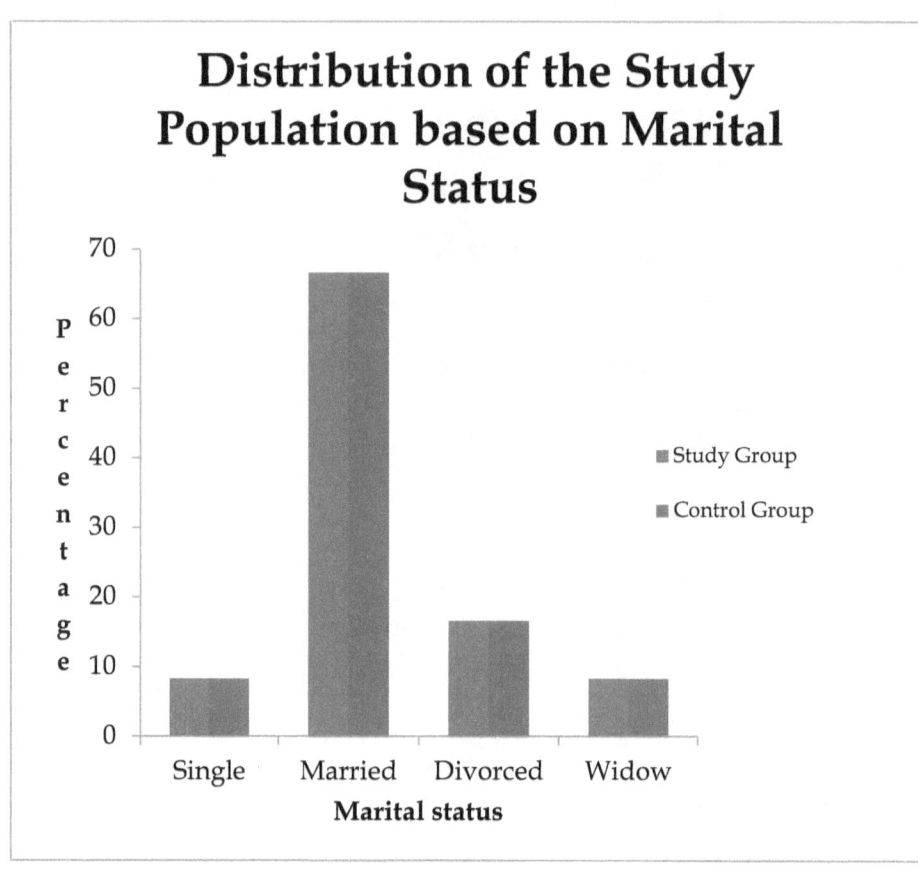

Table 1.6 Distribution of the study population based on the place of residence

Place of Residence	Study group (Frequency)	Study group (Percentage)	Control group (Frequency)	Control group (Percentage)	Total (Frequency)
Nyaruguru District	12	100	12	100	24
Total	12	100	12	100	24

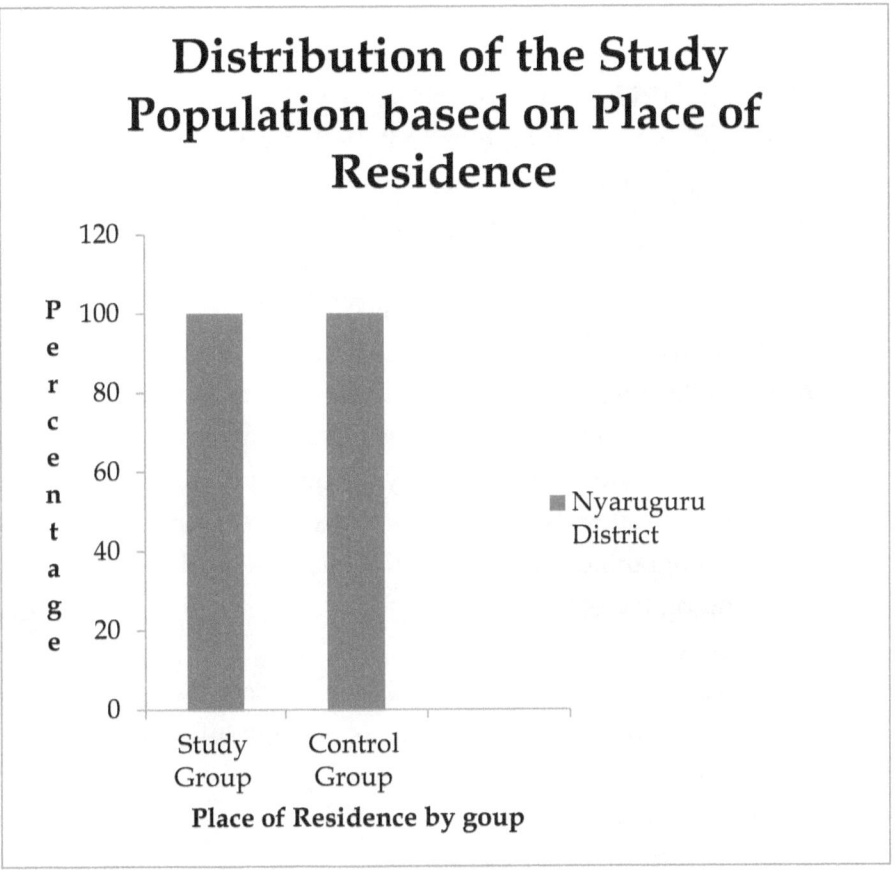

Distribution of the Study Population based on Place of Residence

When I was with a colleague who studied clinical research in the United States of America with much knowledge of statistics especially the STATA software, I requested him to verify the similarity of the study and control groups using the STATA software. I asked him to verify the similarity of the two groups in terms of socio-demographic characteristics such as age. It was not necessary to verify the similarity about the place of residence because all the participants were living in the same place, which was the

NYARUGURU district; or the sex because the number of males and females was the same in both groups.

The study and control groups were similar in terms of marital status because each group had one participant who was single, eight who were married, two who were divorced and one who was a widow.

The two groups were similar in terms of the profession and level of education because all the participants were farmers and no one among all the participants had a level of education superior to the primary school level. I wanted to verify if the study and control groups were similar in all socio-demographic characteristics then exclude any confounding factors.

" ...In the oldest and most widespread usage, confounding is a source of bias in estimating causal effects. This bias is sometimes informally described as mixing of effects of extraneous factors (called confounders) with the effect of interest. This usage predominates in non experimental research, especially in epidemiology and sociology. In a second and more recent usage originating in statistics, confounding is a synonym for change in an effect measure upon stratification or adjustment for extraneous factors (a phenomenon called non collapsibility or Simpson's paradox)."

On the other hand, not only I wanted to exclude any differences about socio-demographic characteristics but also clinical differences had to be excluded between the study and control groups. My colleague told me that by using the STATA software in verifying if there was a difference between the study and control groups, P value had to be superior to 0.05 ($P > 0.05$).

Beginning with the age based on the mean and standard deviation of the study and control groups, he used the T-test by the STATA software because age is a continuous variable. He found that the mean was about forty-one for the study group and forty-two for the control group and the standard deviation was about eight for the study group while the standard deviation was eleven for the control group and P was 0.78866 (P>0.05). So there was no difference of age statistically between the study and control groups; then there was no possible confounding factor to the results due to the age.

Table 1.7 Value of Mean, Standard Deviation and P relating to the Age by group

. ttest age, by(group)

Two-sample t test with equal variances

Group	Obs	Mean	Std. Err.	Std. Dev.	[95% Conf. Interval]	
1	12	40.66667	2.349511	8.138945	35.49543	45.83791
2	12	41.75	3.179301	11.01342	34.75241	48.74759
combined	24	41.20833	1.936472	9.486738	37.20244	45.21423
diff		-1.083333	3.953246		-9.281864	7.115198

diff = mean(1) - mean(2)   t = -0.2740
Ho: diff = 0   degrees of freedom =   22

Ha: diff < 0   Ha: diff != 0   Ha: diff > 0
Pr(T < t) = 0.3933   Pr(|T| > |t|) = 0.7866   Pr(T > t) = 0.6067

Clinically, my colleague started by verifying if there was a difference between the study and control groups about their CD4 by using a T test of the STATA software. We found that the mean of CD4 for the study group was about three hundred and thirty-one and for the control group, the mean was about three hundred and twenty-nine while P was

0.9640 (P>0.05). So there was no difference of CD4 statistically between the study and control groups. Then there was no possible confounding factor to the results due to CD4 count by group.

Table 1.8 Value of Mean, Standard Deviation and P relating to the CD4 count by group

```
. ttest cd4i, by(group)

Two-sample t test with equal variances
```

Group	Obs	Mean	Std. Err.	Std. Dev.	[95% Conf. Interval]	
1	12	331.4167	32.91989	114.0378	258.9605	403.8729
2	12	329.3333	31.62142	109.5398	259.7351	398.9316
combined	24	330.375	22.3228	109.3589	284.1968	376.5532
diff		2.083333	45.64683		-92.5824	96.74907

```
      diff = mean(1) - mean(2)                         t =   0.0456
Ho: diff = 0                          degrees of freedom =       22

   Ha: diff < 0              Ha: diff != 0               Ha: diff > 0
 Pr(T < t) = 0.5180    Pr(|T| > |t|) = 0.9640    Pr(T > t) = 0.4820
```

Using a non parametric test, which is Mann-Whitney or Wilcoxon rank-sum test about viral load, we found that rank sum for the study group was one hundred and sixty and one hundred and forty for the control group while P was 0.4479 (P>0.05). There was no statistically significant difference about viral load at enrollment between the study and control groups. Then there was no possible confounding factor to the results due to viral load by group.

Table 1.9 Value of rank sum based on the viral load by group

```
. ranksum vli, by(group)

Two-sample Wilcoxon rank-sum (Mann-Whitney) test

       group |      obs    rank sum    expected
-------------+---------------------------------
           1 |       12         160         150
           2 |       12         140         150
-------------+---------------------------------
    combined |       24         300         300

unadjusted variance        300.00
adjustment for ties       -126.39
                          ---------
adjusted variance          173.61

Ho: vli(group==1) = vli(group==2)
             z =    0.759
    Prob > |z| =    0.4479

.
```

As results at the end of the study on CD4, we had twelve people living with HIV, in the study group, and three of them equivalent to twenty-five percent had beyond 500 CD4/mm^3, seven of them, equivalent to fifty-eight percent, had from 350 up to 500 CD4/mm^3 and two participants, equivalent to seventeen percent, had between 200 and 349 CD4/mm^3. No one had less than 200 CD4/mm^3 at the end of the study.

Three participants who had more than 500 CD4/mm^3 , precisely for the first one, she had 621 CD4/mm^3 while at the beginning of the study she had had 475 CD4/mm^3. So she had an increase of 146 CD4/mm^3 within three months. For the second one, she had 600 CD4/mm^3 at the end of three months while she had had 304 CD4/mm^3 at the beginning of the study equivalent to an increase of 296 CD4/mm^3 and the third one had 587 CD4/mm^3 at the end

91

of the study while he had had 400 CD4/mm^3 at the beginning equivalent to an increase of 187 CD4/mm^3 within three months.

Seven people living with HIV who had from 350 up to 500 CD4/mm^3 at the end of the study had had less CD4 at the beginning of the study. One of them had 484 CD4/mm^3 from 458 CD4/mm^3, which is equivalent to an increase of 26 CD4/mm^3; the second one had 398 CD4/mm^3 from 340 CD4/mm^3, which is equivalent to an increase of 58 CD4/mm^3 within three months.

On the other hand, one participant in the study group had 369 CD4/mm^3 at the end of the study while he had had 78 CD4/mm^3 at the beginning equivalent to an increase of 291 CD4/mm^3 within only three months just to name but a few.

One participant in the study group with CD4 between 200 and 349 CD4/mm^3 had 294 CD4/mm^3 at the end of the study from 175 CD4/mm^3, which is equivalent to an increase of 119 CD4/mm^3 within three months.

The mean of CD4 at the beginning was 331.4167 CD4/mm^3 and the standard deviation was 114.0378 while at the end of the study the mean of CD4 became 451.4167 CD4/mm^3 and standard deviation to become 106.4651 for the study group.

On average there was an increase of 120 CD4/mm^3 in three months for the study group.

In the control group, we had twelve people living with HIV. No one had beyond 500 CD4/mm^3. Three participants who were equivalent to twenty-five percent had from 350 CD4/mm^3 up to 500 CD4/mm^3. Eight participants who were equivalent to sixty-seven percent had from 200 CD4/mm^3 up to 349 CD4/mm^3 and one participant in the control group who was equivalent to eight percent had less than 200 CD4/mm^3.

Among those who had from 350 CD4/mm^3 up to 500 CD4/mm^3, there were those who had a decrease of CD4 at the end of the study if compared to their CD4 at the beginning of the study. There was one who had 365 CD4/mm^3 at the end from 424 CD4/mm^3 at the beginning of the study and it was equivalent to a decrease of 59 CD4/mm^3 within three months.

Among those who had between 200 and 349 CD4/mm^3, one participant had 314 CD4/mm^3 at the end from 328 CD4/mm^3 at the beginning of the study. Furthermore, in the same interval from 200 CD4/mm^3 up to below 349 CD4/mm^3, there were others who had a decrease of CD4 at the end of the study if compared to their CD4 at the beginning of the study. There was one participant who had 213 CD4/mm^3 at the end of the study from 274 CD4/mm^3 at the beginning of the study, equivalent to a decrease of 61 CD4/mm^3 within three months. Another one had 278 CD4/mm^3 at the end of the study from 375 CD4/mm^3 at the beginning of the study equivalent to a decrease of 97 CD4/mm^3 to name but a few.

Participants in the control group who had below 200CD4/mm^3 got 65 CD4/mm^3 at the end of the study from 67 CD4/mm^3 at the beginning equivalent to a decrease of 2 CD4/mm^3 within three months.

The mean of CD4 at the beginning was 329.3333 CD4/mm^3 with standard deviation of 109.5398 while at the end of the study the mean was 300.0833 CD4/mm^3 with the standard deviation of 101.13673 and on average there was a decrease of 29 CD4/mm^3 in three months for the control group.

Table 2.1 Distribution of the study population based on CD4 at the beginning of the study

CD4/mm^3	Study group (Frequency)	Study group (Percentage)	Control group (Frequency)	Study group (Percentage)	Total
<200	2	16.6	1	8.33	3
200-349	4	33.3	6	50	10
350-500	6	50	5	41.6	11
>500	0	0	0	0	0
Total	12	100	12	100	24

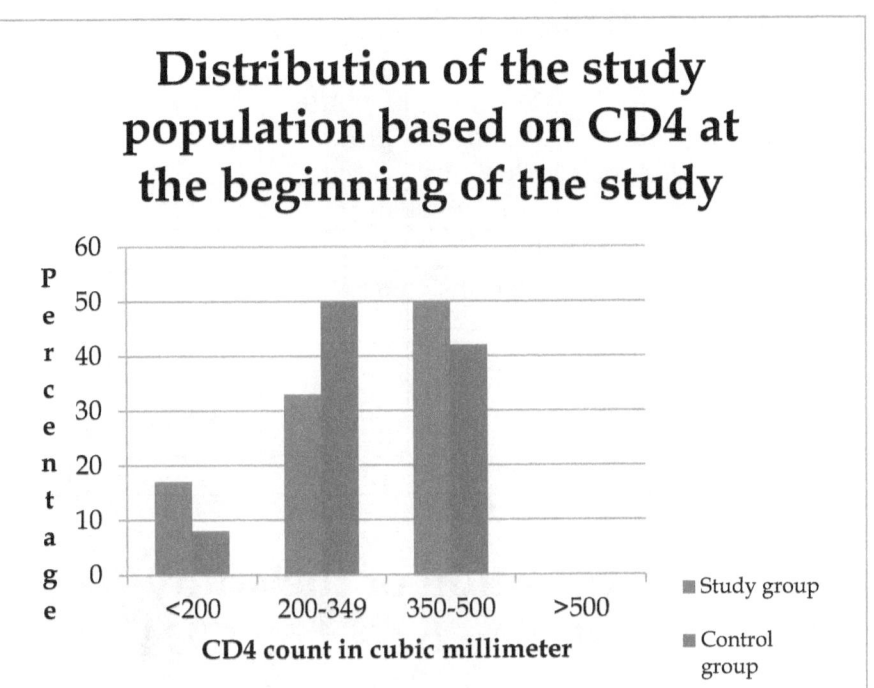

Table 2.2 Distribution of the study population based on CD4 at the end of the study

CD4/mm^3	Study group (Frequency)	Study group (Percentage)	Control group (Frequency)	Study group (Percentage)	Total
<200	0	0	1	8.33	1
200-349	2	16.6	8	66.6	10
350-500	7	58.3	3	25	10
>500	3	25	0	0	3
Total	12	100	12	100	24

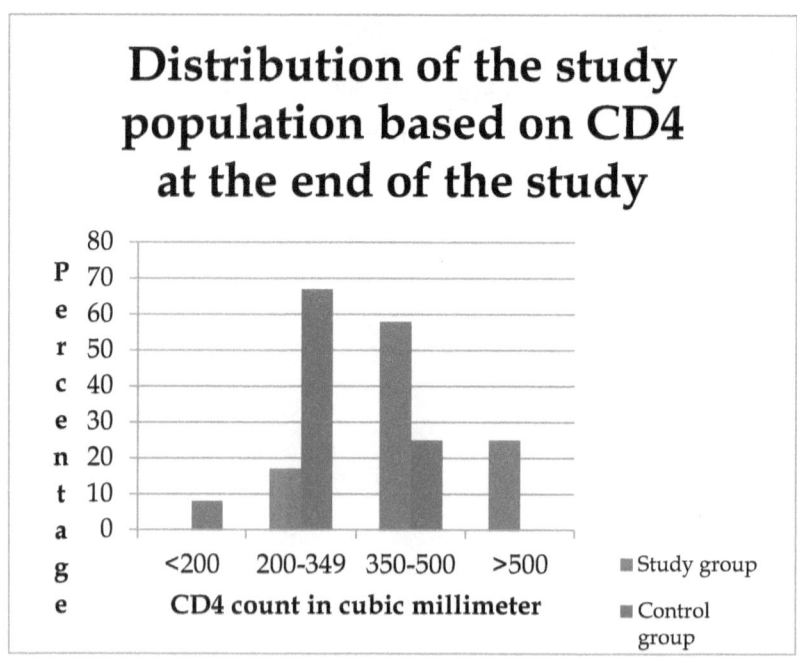

Distribution of the study population based on CD4 at the end of the study

Table 2.3 Value of Mean, Standard Deviation and P relating to CD4 by group
(P<0.05 for the study group)

```
. by group, sort : ttest cd4i == cd4ii
```

```
-> group = 1
```

Paired t test

Variable	Obs	Mean	Std. Err.	Std. Dev.	[95% Conf. Interval]	
cd4i	12	331.4167	32.91989	114.0378	258.9605	403.8729
cd4ii	12	451.4167	30.73382	106.4651	383.772	519.0613
diff	12	-120	27.83474	96.42237	-181.2638	-58.73615

```
    mean(diff) = mean(cd4i - cd4ii)                          t = -4.3112
Ho: mean(diff) = 0                           degrees of freedom =      11

Ha: mean(diff) < 0          Ha: mean(diff) != 0          Ha: mean(diff) > 0
Pr(T < t) = 0.0006        Pr(|T| > |t|) = 0.0012         Pr(T > t) = 0.9994
```

```
-> group = 2
```

Paired t test

Variable	Obs	Mean	Std. Err.	Std. Dev.	[95% Conf. Interval]	
cd4i	12	329.3333	31.62142	109.5398	259.7351	398.9316
cd4ii	12	300.0833	29.19565	101.1367	235.8242	364.3425
diff	12	29.25	15.3357	53.12443	-4.503649	63.00365

```
    mean(diff) = mean(cd4i - cd4ii)                          t =  1.9073
Ho: mean(diff) = 0                           degrees of freedom =      11

Ha: mean(diff) < 0          Ha: mean(diff) != 0          Ha: mean(diff) > 0
Pr(T < t) = 0.9585        Pr(|T| > |t|) = 0.0829         Pr(T > t) = 0.0415
```

For viral load, in the study group, we had twelve people living with HIV and nine of them equivalent to seventy-five percent had viral load below 20 RNA copies/ml and two participants who were equivalent to seventeen percent had viral load below 20 Log 1.30 RNA copies/ml and one participant who was equivalent to eight percent had viral load below 1.50 RNA copies/ml at the end of the study.

All twelve people living with HIV who had below 20 RNA copies/ml at the end of the study, most of them had had viral load below 20 RNA copies/ml at the beginning of the study but there were four who had 20 RNA copies/ml at the beginning of the study. One participant who had had viral load equivalent to 65.4 Log 1.82 RNA copies/ml at the beginning, had a change that was measured and he had below 20 Log 1.30 RNA copies/ml at the end of the study. For that participant, in the study group, it was possible to observe a decrease of viral load from the beginning up to the end of the study because 65.4 Log 1.82 RNA copies/ml was superior to 20 Log 1.30 copies/ml.

We could not know what represented viral load below 20 RNA copies/ml as such a result was undetectable. So it was impossible to know if below 20 RNA copies/ml was 0 RNA copy/ml or 1 RNA copy/ml or more for instance 19 RNA copies/ml. So we could not use any statistical method by STATA software because viral load below 20 RNA copies/ml was not defined and no correct figure could replace it.

However a decrease of viral load was observed in the study group for example the one who came from viral load of 65.4 Log 1.82 RNA copies/ml at the beginning of the study up to viral load that was below 20 Log 1.30 RNA copies/ml at the end of the study.

In the control group, we had twelve people living with HIV and seven of them equivalent to fifty eight percent had viral load below 20 RNA copies/ml at the end of the study. Three of them equivalent to twenty-five percent had viral load below 20 Log 1.30 RNA copies/ml at the end of the study. Two participants who were equivalent to seventeen percent had viral load of 20 RNA copies/ml at the end of the study. We could not know the correct figure representing viral load below 20 RNA copies/ml and it was not possible to use any statistical methods by the STATA software. However an increase of viral load in the control group at the end of the study was observed for instance the one who came from viral load of 856 Log 2.93 RNA copies/ml at the beginning of the study up to 84,000 Log 4.92 RNA copies/ml at the end of the study within three months equivalent to an increase of about 83,144 RNA copies/ml.

Table 2.3 Distribution of the study population based on viral load at the beginning of the study

Viral load (RNA copies/ml)	Study group (Frequency)	Study group (Percentage)	Control group (Frequency)	Control group (Percentage)	Total (Frequency)
<20	8	67	10	83	18
>20	4	33	2	17	6
Total	12	100	12	100	24

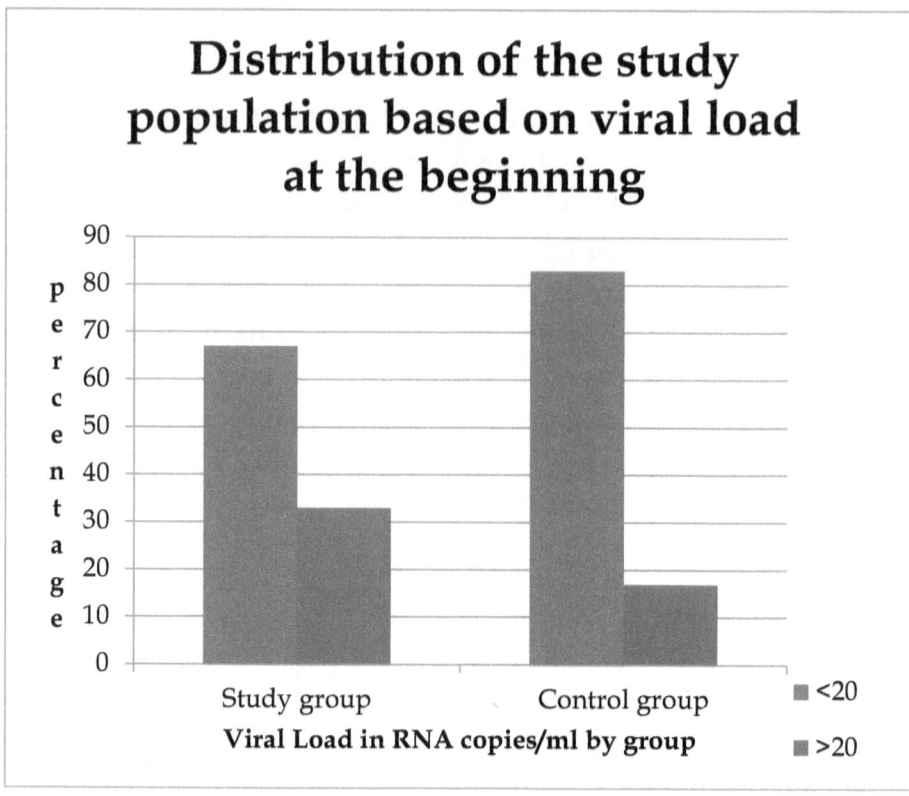

Table 2.4 Distribution of the study population based on viral load at the end of the study

Viral load (RNA copies/ ml)	Study group (Freque ncy)	Study group (Percent age)	Control group (Freque ncy)	Control group (Percent age)	Total (Freque ncy)
<20	12	100	9	75	21
>20	0	0	3	25	3
Total	12	100	12	100	24

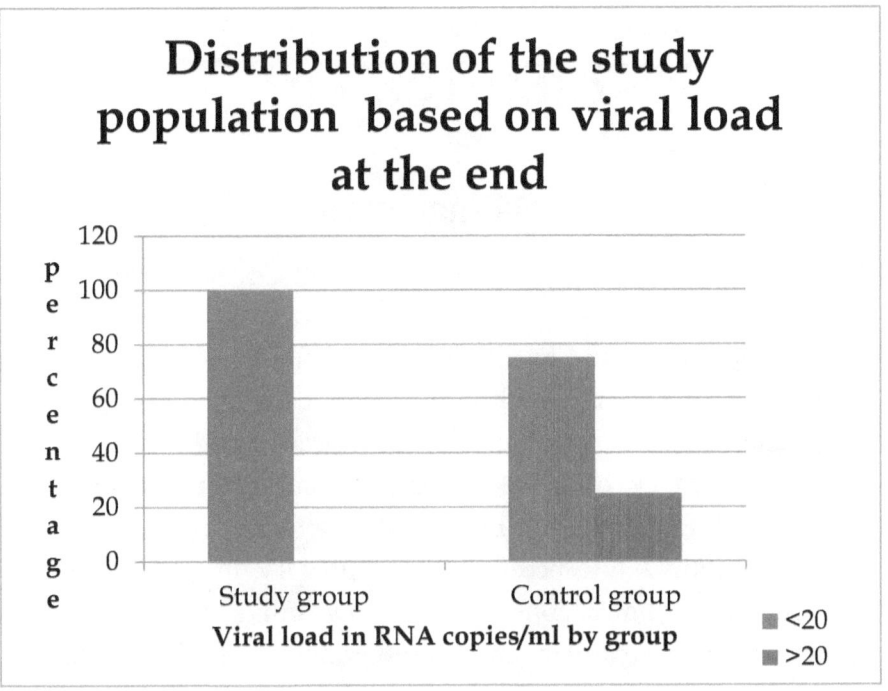

CHAPTER XII

CD4 increased

On CD4, the results were good. People living with HIV, in the study group, who consumed one liter of cow milk per day for three months had an increase of CD4 of about one hundred and twenty CD4 per cubic millimeter (120 CD4/mm^3) on average within only three months while people living with HIV in the control group who didn't consume the cow milk within three months in the similar socio-demographic conditions with similar characteristics like the participants in the study group, had a decrease of CD4 of about twenty-nine CD4 per cubic millimeter (29 CD4/mm^3).

The results showed that there was a significant association statistically between consuming the cow milk and a rapid increase of CD4 with threshold $\alpha=0.05$, P=0.0012.

Several studies have been done in the United States of America, China, Sweden and the Netherlands whereby different proteins of the cow milk showed that they were inhibitors of human immunodeficiency virus type 1 (HIV1).

In the cow milk, there is a protein called lactoferrin that prevents the transmission of HIV1 by the dendritic cells, which are normally able to keep HIV1 for some days and transmit it to CD4. The lactoferrin inhibits strongly the reverse transcriptase of HIV1, inhibits not strongly the protease and integrase of HIV1. The lactoferrin is bound to V3 of the gp120, which is one of the proteins of HIV envelop.

Three other proteins of the cow milk, alpha lactalbumin, beta lactoglobulin and casein inhibit the protease and the integrase of HIV1 sufficiently but don't inhibit the reverse transcriptase.

Other two proteins of the cow milk, which are glycolactin and angiogenin-1 inhibit moderately the activity of the reverse transcriptase of HIV1, inhibit strongly the protease and the integrase of HIV1. In comparison with other proteins of the cow milk, the glycolactin is the strongest inhibitor of the protease and the integrase but moderate inhibitor of the reverse transcriptase of HIV1.

Another protein of the cow milk is lactogenin. It is a strong inhibitor of the integrase, moderate inhibitor of the reverse transcriptase and weak inhibitor of the protease of HIV1.

The lactoperoxidase is another protein of the cow milk and it inhibits the activity of the reverse transcriptase of HIV1.

On the other hand, the cow milk is a complete nutrient for a human being and it has water (90%), proteins (3-4g/100g), carbohydrates (4.8-5.2/100g), fat (3.5-6g/100g), minerals like potassium (138mg/100ml), calcium (125mg/100ml), chlorine (103mg/100ml), phosphorus (96mg/100ml), sodium (50mg/100ml), sulfur (30mg/100ml), magnesium (12mg/100ml), micro minerals including cobalt, copper, iron (0.1mg/100g), manganese, molybdenum, zinc, selenium, iodine (22mg/l), and vitamins like vitamin A (39μg/100g), vitamin B1 (0.05mg/100g), vitamin B12 (0.17mg/100g), vitamin C (0.6mg/100g), vitamin D (0.03μg/100g), vitamin E (0.07mg/100g), vitamin PP-

Pellagra Preventing Factor or Nicotinamide (0.16mg/100g), vitamin B5 (0.35mg/100g), vitamin B9 (3µg/100g), vitamin K1 (17µg/dl), folic acid (37.7µg/dl), osmotic concentration (23mOsm/dl). The cow milk has 750 kilocalories/liter.

For our study, considering the capacity of the cow milk with proteins that inhibit HIV1 and based on how the cow milk is a complete nutrient, we contributed to solve a problem of a low CD4 increase for people living with HIV on ART who are poor.

When I was in medicine, I studied infectious diseases including HIV. I learned in that course that someone who is HIV positive, on antiretroviral treatment, can have his or her viral load decreased and CD4 increased and the maximum increase of CD4 in six months was about one hundred CD4 per cubic millimeter (100 CD4/mm^3). I realized that what I learned in theory was true when I started clinical practices in third year of medicine called doctorate I, whereby so many people living with HIV came to the hospital of the University of Rwanda in BUTARE to be hospitalized. I remember that the majority of them had a decrease of CD4 leading them to opportunistic infections such as pulmonary tuberculosis, pneumonia and meningitis to name but a few. Those infections used to kill so many patients and it was a big issue in medicine and in our hospital because a big number of deaths were due to HIV/AIDS.

Even those who had an increase of CD4, no one had an increase of CD4 of more than one hundred CD4 per cubic millimeter (100CD4/mm^3) in six months despite the antiretroviral treatment taken. I could find some people living with HIV with an increase of their CD4 from

$150CD4/mm^3$ to $190CD4/mm^3$ within six months and as I learned in medicine CD4 below $500/mm^3$ was a risk of opportunistic infections especially for poor people.

When there was a risk of opportunistic infections, there was also a risk of death. That is why I started to think what I could do to contribute in solving that problem and in 2008, I did a study whereby I observed for my first time a rapid increase of CD4 about $100CD4/mm^3$ on average in three months only. I remember that one of the participants had an increase of CD4 of two hundred and fifty $CD4/mm^3$ $(250CD4/mm^3)$ in three months just because of consuming the cow milk during three month period of time.

People who had a rapid increase of CD4 didn't have opportunistic infections and there was no high risk of death. They were discharged without staying for a long time in the hospital and this situation had clinical and economic impacts. Clinically, when a patient is discharged without staying for a long time in a hospital especially the one living with HIV with a low immunity and he or she avoids many nosocomial infections, which have a resistance to different drugs.

"Nosocomial infections are infections that were not present before the patient came to a hospital, but were acquired by a patient while in the hospital. Mentioned in enterobacterial infections, staphylococcal infections."

I remember that at Kigali University Teaching hospital, in internal medicine department, in 2008, there were so many patients who had different pathologies such as pulmonary tuberculosis, pneumonia, meningitis, Kaposi's sarcoma to name but a few. Among patients living with HIV who were hospitalized in the internal medicine department, some had pulmonary tuberculosis, others meningitis at admission and according to hospitalization for a long period of time, while staying in the hospital, one could have meningitis at admission and pulmonary tuberculosis during his or her hospitalization. If the discharge was done very quickly, the risk of having more nosocomial infections could have been decreased. The risk of deaths among those who left the hospital rapidly was decreased too.

On the other hand, economically, there is an impact when a patient is discharged quickly because he or she pays to the hospital not as much money as that has to be paid by someone who stays for a long period of time in a hospital. The family of an hospitalized patient has to spend a lot of money in travelling while members of his or her family are coming to visit him or her but also in buying what has been requested by their patient. Furthermore, there is no productivity for a patient who is hospitalized.

I remember at Kigali University Teaching hospital where there were many patients living with HIV who had to stay at the hospital for some months while on treatment. They had to be fed by their families because the ministry of health in Rwanda was offering some nutritional support to indigents living with HIV but at only 60% of their needs in energy. So the support was not enough and their families had to find the remaining 40% of their daily needs in terms of energy. Those hospitalized patients could not work and not only they needed a nutritional support from their families but also in terms of hygiene they were in need of for example a soap, tooth brush and tooth paste, from their families. So economically, their families had to pay a lot of money due to their needs and the expenses increased when their relatives stayed for a long period of time in the hospital. For those who consumed one liter of cow milk per day for three months, their CD4 were increased rapidly and they didn't have a lot of opportunistic infections and they were discharged very quickly, which allowed them to decrease the expenses for their families and themselves. Moreover, when patients were discharged very quickly, they went home where some of them found jobs that allowed them to increase their income for them and their families.

So the study helped the patients in the study group clinically but also economically.

On viral load, in the study done at the MUNINI hospital, the results were characterized by a laboratory limitation in measuring viral load below 20 RNA copies/ml.

However a decreased viral load was observed for people living with HIV who consumed the cow milk while an increased viral load was noticed in the control group. Viral load below 20 RNA copies/ml is called undetectable and the TAQMAN system could not differentiate 0 RNA copy/ml, 1 RNA copy/ml and 2 RNA copies/ml up to 19 RNA copies/ml. Some patients had had viral load below 20 RNA copies/ml at the beginning of the study and they had the same viral load below 20 RNA copies/ml at the end of the study.

So we were not able to determine the correct figure representing viral load below 20 RNA copies/ml and it was not possible to use any statistical methods by the STATA software.

However just as an example, a patient in the study group, had had viral load of 65.4Log1.82 RNA copies/ml at the beginning of the study and at the end of the study, that patient had viral load below 20 RNA copies/ml, which was a decreased viral load at a point of having undetectable viral load.

On the contrary, just as an example, a patient in the control group, had had viral load of 856Log2.93 RNA copies/ml at the beginning of the study and that patient had viral load of 84,000Log4.92 RNA copies/ml at the end of the study, which was an increased viral load at the end of the study.

Again I remember that different studies in developed countries such as the United states of America, Sweden, the Netherlands and in China have shown that in cow milk there were inhibitors of human immunodeficiency virus type 1 (HIV1). In the cow milk, the first protein is called lactoferrin and it prevents the transmission of HIV1 by the dendritic cells, which are normally able to keep HIV1 for some days and transmit it to CD4. The lactoferrin inhibits strongly the reverse transcriptase of HIV1, inhibits but not strongly the protease and integrase of HIV1. The lactoferrin is bound to V3 of the gp 120, which is one of the proteins of HIV envelop.

There are three other proteins of the cow milk, which are alpha lactalbumin, beta lactoglobulin and casein. They inhibit the protease and the integrase of HIV1 sufficiently but don't inhibit the reverse transcriptase.

Other two proteins of the cow milk which are glycolactin and angiogenin-1. They inhibit moderately the activity of the reverse transcriptase of HIV1, inhibit strongly the protease and the integrase of HIV1.

In comparison with other proteins of the cow milk, the glycolactin is the strongest inhibitor of the protease and integrase but moderate inhibitor of the reverse transcriptase of HIV1. Another protein of the cow milk is lactogenin. It is a strong inhibitor of the integrase, moderate inhibitor of the reverse transcriptase and weak inhibitor of the protease of HIV1. Finally, the lactoperoxidase is another protein of the cow milk and it inhibits the activity of the reverse transcriptase of HIV1.

For our study, considering the capacity of the cow milk with its proteins that inhibit HIV1, we contributed to solve a problem of an increase of viral load for some patients living with HIV while they were on ART.

In conclusion, the hypothesis was confirmed. As the hypothesis was "The cow milk increases CD4 of people living with HIV", we saw that the results were good because people living with HIV, in the study group, who consumed one liter of cow milk per day for three months had an increase of CD4 of about one hundred and twenty CD4 per cubic millimeter (120 CD4/mm^3) on average within only three months, while people living with HIV in the control group who didn't consume the cow milk within three months and living in the similar socio-demographic conditions with similar clinical characteristics like participants in the study group, had a decrease of CD4 of about twenty-nine CD4 per cubic millimeter (29 CD4/mm^3) at the MUNINI hospital.

The results showed that there was a significant association statistically between consuming the cow milk and rapid increase of CD4 with a threshold $\alpha=0.05$, $P=0.0012$.

On the other hand, with regard viral load, the results were characterized by a laboratory limitation in measuring viral load below 20 RNA copies/ml. However a decrease of viral load was observed for people living with HIV who consumed the cow milk while an increase of viral load was noticed in the control group.

One of the recommendations was that people living with HIV should consume one liter of cow milk per day for three months to increase rapidly their CD4.

Another recommendation was that another study should be done on a large sample size.

CHAPTER XIII

My work in a remote hospital

The remote hospital is called MUNINI hospital. It is located in the southern province of Rwanda at about 165Kms or 103 miles from Kigali, the capital city. It is in the district of NYARUGURU. This district has a place called KIBEHO where has been apparition of the Virgin Mary, the mother of Jesus Christ, in the 1980s. It is the only approved holy land in Africa and other holy lands are on other continents especially Europe at Lourdes and Fatima according to the Roman Catholic Church. I remember that I met one of the girls who had had apparition and who still lived at KIBEHO in 2015. It was on Assumption of Mary 2015 or August 15, 2015 when I was at KIBEHO with a medical team. This team had a medical doctor, anesthetist, a nurse and a mental health nurse as well as a driver plus an ambulance, from MUNINI hospital to solve all health problems during that important event. Many people came during such an event and they were mainly Christians of Roman Catholic Church from Rwanda but also from other countries such as Rwanda neighboring countries: Uganda, Democratic Republic of Congo, Tanzania, Burundi and around the world: from the United States of America, Poland to name but a few. They were estimated at around 25,000 people and some of them came in what they called a holy walk to the holy place far from where they lived. Many People came to KIBEHO by foot from several places of Rwanda including the capital city of Kigali and others from abroad. An example is a man who came from Uganda by foot and he had left his country, Poland, some days ago for that holy walk from Kampala to KIBEHO. It was an incredible example of a courageous Christian with a strong belief, indeed. Those who came by foot spent their nights on a way to the holy land and slept at any places in that way including the sides of roads. Many of them spent about three days and nights to reach the place and they were tired and some had hypoglycemia and dizziness and a few could be in coma. Not only there was a medical team but also there were essential drugs including glucose, from MUNINI hospital, to allow the team to manage such fatal cases without any problems. Those people who were in coma due to hypoglycemia were given glucose, they were no longer in that status after getting glucose and they became normal. There were many musculoskeletal diseases due to a big distance done in their walk before reaching the Holy land and all those cases were properly managed. Some complicated cases needed a thorough follow-up and admission in a nearby health center. Those complicated cases were especially severe malaria with high profuse sweating, fever of 39 up to 40 degree Celsius, headache, nausea, vomiting and abdominal pain to name but a few. The rapid test of malaria was positive and a blood sample was taken for blood smear and a treatment of severe malaria was initiated and a concerned patient was kept in a room for emergency cases while trying to stabilize him or her. After stabilization, the patient was admitted in a nearby health center for further treatment, which was well specified for the health center. No one died, during such a huge event, due to any causes of death and that success was due to a good and quick management of all cases. As I was on site, I went to see one of the girls who had had apparition of the Virgin Mary. She was the only girl who was still living at the holy land of KIBEHO in Rwanda. After knocking on a door of her house, I waited for a while and when I opened the door, I found that it was not locked. She came directly from her room to welcome me in her sitting room. I introduced myself and she told me she had felt someone was coming to visit her. She continued by telling me that it was not usual to have the feeling that brought her to let her house's door, not locked, which was normally locked unless an appointment was given by herself. She told me she was called Mukampazimpaka Natalie and was 50. She could tell me that she had apparition of Virgin Mary in 1982 when she was in fourth year of high school. That high school is the one located at KIBEHO near her house. Virgin Mary apparitions happened to two more girls who were her colleagues at the high school. Those two girls were Mumureke Alphonsine who started to get apparition of Virgin Mary in 1981 and Mukangango Marie Claire who was the third girl to have apparitions in 1982 after Natalie. She told me that Virgin Mary mentioned to her that people were committing many sins and they were betraying each other at a high level without love between them but with selfishness. Virgin Mary continued to tell Natalie that such attitudes were not making happy God and people should stop such bad behaviors. Furthermore, Virgin Mary told Natalie that she would convey such a message to all people around her and stay at KIBEHO for that purpose. Natalie told me that she was not allowed to leave that place according to what Virgin Mary told her. Mukampazimpaka Natalie remembered that one time in one of apparitions, Virgin Mary who was very angry and while crying, told her that there were going to happen many killings in Rwanda. Many Rwandans, including children and women, were going to be killed and among their killers, mainly, they would be other Rwandans. So, Rwandans were going to be killed by a majority of killers who would be Rwandans. Rwandan blood was going to flow and mass graves, in Rwanda, were going to be full of dead bodies. Natalie was first of all afraid when she saw Virgin Mary in a different appearance and secondly afraid of what she heard from her and that would happen to Rwandans in Rwanda. When Genocide happened in 1994, Natalie remembered that Virgin Mary had already told her about it and saw killings of children, women among others; blood flowing; mass graves and many dead bodies inside them similar to what she had known before in the above mentioned apparition.

I asked Natalie what she had learned from Virgin Mary. Mukampazimpaka Natalie told me that she learned from Virgin Mary that selfishness and betrayal were very bad and must be avoided by people in this world because even God doesn't like them. Another thing she could learn from Virgin Mary was how to speak quietly. My second question was how she solved her family problems financially. She told me that her father was living at MUNINI sector where is located the MUNINI hospital. She mentioned that her father had died and she prayed and some sponsors helped her for her father's burial events. She told me that for each family problem she normally prays and a solution is found from people who helped her. She also mentioned that the

Catholic Church helps her in terms of feeding, housing and paying for needs in health in case she is sick, just to name as examples. She told me that her disease was dental and she normally consulted dentists in the capital city of Rwanda, Kigali. She gave me her phone number and I gave her mine and I promised her that in case she needed my help especially in terms of disease management I would be there to help her.

After my study of medicine at the National University of Rwanda, now the University of Rwanda, at the end of 2008, I was called to work in KANOMBE hospital, which is one of the biggest hospitals in Rwanda and that hospital is located in Kigali. While I was waiting for my graduation ceremony, I started to work in KANOMBE hospital on January 1, 2009 as head of out-patient and emergency department, which was one of the busiest departments in that hospital. I was committed to work very hard and to save as many lives as possible. At that time, there was not a hospital in the rest of the KICUKIRO district, yet. KICUKIRO district, which is one of the three districts in the Kigali city, didn't have a district hospital in 2009 and all health centers in that district used to transfer patients to KANOMBE hospital. That district has $167Km^2$ of total surface area, a population of about 318,564 according to 2012 Census, 10 sectors and 10 health centers. Those sectors are: Niboye, Kagarama, Kicukiro, Kanombe, Nyarugunga, Gikondo, Kigarama, Gatenga, Gahanga and Masaka. Health Centers are: Kicukiro located at Niboye sector, Betsaida located at Kicukiro sector, Gikondo located at Gikondo sector, Nyarugunga located at Nyarugunga Sector, Busanza located at Kanombe sector,

Kairos located at Kanombe sector, Gatenga located at Gatenga sector, Gahanga located at Gahanga sector, Masaka located at Masaka sector and Kabuga located at Masaka sector. All people of Kicukiro district who consulted the health centers in that district used to be transferred to Kanombe hospital because the district hospital of Kicukiro, which is the Masaka hospital, was not there in 2009. Many patients came to the out-patient and emergency department if compared to patients who went to other departments at the Kanombe hospital. Not only patients who were transferred from Kicukiro district health centers but also patients with insurances, allowing them to consult directly without waiting for a transfer, consulted Kanombe hospital. An example of such insurances is a health insurance for public servants provided by Rwanda Social Security Board (RSSB). Private patients without any insurances, and all emergency cases used to be managed at Kanombe hospital, especially the Out-patient and emergency department, which was managing the majority of cases. I worked very hard and I could have around 80 patients, in consultation per day, who were all receiving an appropriate treatment. I decided to work without going to a break at lunch time and I could deliver a quick and adequate treatment to each and every patient consulting the out-patient and emergency department of Kanombe hospital. People were very happy of the service delivery offered to them and other patients from other districts or who had started consulting other hospitals, came to the out-patient and emergency department of Kanombe hospital in particular. I remember one patient who phoned me from Texas in the United States of America saying that he was thankful for the way I had saved his life after having consulted many hospitals without success. I was proud of that message and I knew that my efforts made to save people's lives at Out-patient and emergency department of Kanombe hospital were helpful.

When I was in Kanombe hospital, I went to different missions including the United Nations (UN) peacekeeping mission in Sudan. This mission started in September 2009 and ended in September 2010. It was a one-year UN mission where I had to lead a Rwandan medical team that had several medical doctors, nurses and different health professionals. The preparations started by a training of all concerned persons who would participate in that mission. I had to get a service passport and all medical needs including drugs were ready at the departure for the mission. We took a flight from Kigali to Darfur in Sudan. In the medical department of the mission at my workplace, I was with other two medical doctors and several health professionals including nurses. I remember that we arrived in Darfur in the afternoon and it was very sunny. A large delegation of Rwandans who were there came to welcome us because they had known about our arrival. We went to our workplace, which was called Zamzam in Darfur. There was a level one clinic according to the United Nations classification and it is compared to a health facility where it is delivered primary health care. I could do consultation and minor surgery. There were technicians in anesthesia, laboratory, dental, physiotherapy and mental health departments. Furthermore, there were nurses and I remember that one day one member, of our group at Zamzam, was wounded on his leg. I had to examine him and fortunately, I found that he didn't have a fracture. As I was assisted by experienced nurses, we managed that case, which didn't cause any problems at all. I sent the patient to level two clinic of the United Nations for X-ray check-up. The level two clinic of the United Nations was at El FASHER in Darfur and it had radiography department among other departments. The X-ray showed that there was no fracture as I had already seen it in my examination. Doctors at the level two clinic were very happy about the diagnosis we mentioned for the patient and our management of the case. They started to give us credit for our good case management. As they were normally our referral health facility, they were confident of how we were managing cases and our patients would be welcomed to their clinic without delay of too much check-ups on what we would have already done. The level two clinic of the United Nations in Darfur in Sudan had many departments including surgery, dental, laboratory and radiography departments to name but a few. In those departments, the clinic had competent staff and adequate equipment according to the United Nations requirements. They had specialists in surgery, dental, laboratory, radiography and so on and so forth. The head of the United Nations level two clinic in Darfur was a surgeon and he always appreciated how we were managing cases. I remember that some cases for example in dental department were sent to our clinic at Zamzam from the level two clinic, when they had any problems either of equipment or staff, and all those cases were handled appropriately. This brought more insurance to all the staff of that higher clinic in the United Nations and even its leadership was confident that any cases were properly handled at our level one clinic. On the other hand, we had a big issue when it started raining whereby there was standing water at many places around our clinic. We registered many cases of malaria and we used medications against malaria we had at that time including quinine and coartem, which is a combination of artemether and lumefantrine. One tablet of coartem has 20mg of artemether and 120mg of lumefantrine and it is orally consumed. Coartem has shown efficacy in treating malaria in three days according to several studies done especially in Rwanda and it has been approved by the World Health Organization. However, some resistance of malaria against that drug has been mentioned in Asian countries for example in Thailand according to research done in that part of the world. I remember one patient who came to the clinic with asthenia, sweating, saying that he had anorexia and when I measured his temperature he had 39 degree Celsius. In his history, the patient mentioned that he had got some problems when in the past he had been treated by quinine on a malaria case. I thought about malaria for his diagnosis and the blood sample was taken for blood smear. While waiting for result, I intramuscularly gave him an antipyretic to decrease his fever. The result of blood smear confirmed that the patient had malaria. I gave him coartem, which is 20mg artemether and 120mg lumefantrine, 4 tablets times two a day for three days and for the first day the interval, between the first 4 tablets and the second 4 tabs, was eight hours. For the two following days, the interval was twelve hours and the total dosage in 3 days was 24 tablets according to the guideline, as the patient was an adult. After 3 days, the patient could not improve and had the same symptoms and signs he came with the first day of his consultation such as asthenia, sweating and fever among others. I could not give him quinine because he had mentioned problems with it in his past history. I thought it was probably a resistance of his malaria to coartem and I decided to continue giving him that drug. After 5 days, the malaria symptoms and signs for the patient disappeared and I had to confirm such an improvement by a blood smear that was malaria-negative. This is a new and good thing, which shows that changes do exist in science with success especially in terms of saving lives. On the other hand, with the above mentioned example of malaria new treatment guideline, I remember paradigm described on page 26 in the book: "What The Bleep Do We Know" written by William Arntz, Betsy Chasse and Mark Vicente. "A paradigm is like a theory, but a little different...A paradigm, furthermore, is a set of implicit assumptions that are not meant to be tested; in fact they are essentially unconscious." There are many examples even in medicine, which were thought not possible to be changed but, which have changed. Those examples are on cancer and virus to name but a few.

In the past, all cancers were incurable diseases, but now some cancers can be treated and healed when they are diagnosed and treated at an earlier stage. An example of a cancer that can be healed is breast cancer when its treatment is started earlier. Viruses used to kill human beings because there was no remedy, but thinks have now changed. With the research, there are now vaccines and treatments that save human lives. An example of such an important vaccine is the vaccine against measles.

On the other hand, personally, when I studied medicine before my research, it was known that a maximum increase of CD4 for people living with HIV was 100CD4/cubic millimeter in six months even when a patient was on antiretroviral treatment. With my research that was about giving one liter of cow milk, which is a complete nutrient and inhibits HIV, to patients living with HIV in a study group for 3 months, I realized that there was an increase of 120 CD4/cubic millimeter on average in only three months. This was a tremendous improvement in terms of immunity of people living with HIV.

In the United Nations peacekeeping mission in Darfur, I had to appropriately treat many cases of malaria and I had a shortage of drugs to treat that disease because that number of patients was not expected. I had to solve that problem in two ways. One, I had to fumigate with an adequate product against malaria at all places where there were our people. This was a prevention measure because without such a preventive measure, we wouldn't have been able to cope with an increasing number of patients. On the other hand, I had to request more drugs from Rwanda and the response was that I could go myself to bring them to my workplace because there was no schedule of a flight, which would urgently come from Rwanda to Sudan. I was ready and I had to go from Sudan to Uganda with a usual United Nations flight. When I arrived at Entebbe airport, I found another schedule with a Rwandan company "Rwandair" and it had already been paid for my Entebbe-Kigali trip by Rwanda. While waiting for the flight, I visited supermarkets within the Entebbe airport waiting place and I saw a nice telephone. The color of that telephone was red-violet and its cost was $100. As I had that amount of money, I decided to buy it for my wife called Uwimana Jacqueline, as a gift for her, because I had been far from my home for quite some time. I left Entebbe airport at around 6PM local time and arrived in Kigali in the evening and I could only see lights of houses in the capital city of Rwanda, Kigali. My wife came to welcome me at the airport and I gave her the gift. She was surprised, she opened her gift and when she saw that it was a nice telephone, she was very happy. The following day I went to find necessary drugs that would allowed us to pursue our UN peacekeeping mission without any other drug issue. Among needed drugs, there were drugs to treat malaria and I found them all. I had to find a bid bag to transport them from Kigali to Sudan. I took the flight, the third day, from Kigali to Entebbe and when I arrived at Entebbe, I had a problem because the flight from Entebbe to Sudan was not available on time. I was obliged to wait for some two more days when the flight was then available. In the meantime, I had to go to a guest house near the airport for the two days while waiting the flight. When it came, I went to Sudan starting with Juba because South Sudan was still part of Sudan, after Juba the flight went to Khartoum, the capital city of Sudan. In Khartoum, I had to visit our staff and I found them in a good welfare without any particular problems. After Khartoum, I went back to Darfur and particularly ZAMZAM where was my specific workplace. When the staff saw me, they were very happy because they knew that the problem of malaria drug stock-out would not happen again. As soon as I arrived, I sent a message to all medical staff at different areas in the UN peacekeeping mission in Darfur including El FASHER, KABKABIYA and ZARINGE, just as examples, so that they could send a request of the urgent needed drugs from their respective areas. The following day, after getting their requests, I did an allocation according to their needs and I sent the allocated drugs to them. They were very happy, too, because the problem, of not having enough drugs to treat malaria, was solved in their areas. Furthermore, I urged all heads of medical staff in the mission area to do fumigation everywhere it had not been done yet. They did it and with all those mentioned strategies, we could stop the malaria outbreak, in the United Nations peacekeeping mission, without having killed a single person in our different workplaces.

On the other hand, another issue was a risk of having non communicable diseases due to unbalanced diet for many people in the mission. There was a diet of much carbohydrates for example juices and there were many types of juice, in a large quantity, such as apple and mango to name but a few. The diet had much fats too, with chips, eggs and so on and so forth. People started to have an increased weight and I decided to buy weighing scales so that each and every clinic had at least one weighing scale. I began a sensitization so that everyone started to know his/her weight on regular basis at least once a week, therefore his or her body mass index had to be calculated by a health provider based on his or her height and weight. The BMI or Body Mass Index is calculated as follows: Weight in Kilograms divided by the square of the Height in meters. For example if someone has 70Kgs of weight and a height of 1.70m, his or her BMI is $70/(1.70)^2$, which becomes 70/1.70x1.70 or 70/2.89, which is finally 24 Kg/m^2. Note that the normal range is 18.5 Kg/m^2 up to 25 Kg/m^2 according to World Health Organization (WHO). The person who has body mass index (BMI) also called QUETELET index of 24, is in a normal range. Anyone who has a BMI above 25 up to 30, is overweight and above 30, is obese. Those people who have BMI under 18.5 are underweight. People started to have a BMI above 25, which means that they were starting to be overweight and I urged them to increase physical exercises and to get a balanced diet without stopping regular weight check-up. For some months, changes happened and BMI was between 18.5 and 24 for many people, which was normal. I encouraged them to continue doing much physical exercises in particular. However, from three months in the mission, there was a high level of stress because people were far from their country and families. This stress was among causes of non-communicable diseases such as mental health issues, high blood pressure and even diabetes. I remember one patient who consulted with signs of diabetes such as polyuria or production of abnormally large volumes of dilute urine, POLLAKIURIA or abnormally frequent urination and polydipsia, which is a feeling of excessive thirst. The patient came with asthenia or fatigue and an abnormal weight loss. When blood sample was taken for glycemia or sugar in blood, it was found that he had a hyperglycemia and the conclusion was that he had diabetes. We treated him with insuline and after some time he recovered and the glycemia became normal. This showed me that with stress, some people can have a high level of blood sugar or hyperglycemia with all above mentioned signs and symptoms of diabetes. One of the strategies used, were to organize regular training in the afternoon at least 5 days a week. Among topics, there was one on stress and people knew how to manage it. There were other diseases that could kill our people at any time. Those diseases were for example HIV/AIDS. Before going to the mission, I knew those who had such a disease and they had Antiretroviral drugs for at least one month. Once that month was ended, other drugs, for people living with HIV in the mission, were sent from Rwanda. Furthermore, I did a regular follow-up on those people by measuring their vital signs and giving them advice. Among what I urged them to do, there was advice on consuming cow milk daily because it is a new and good drug against HIV/AIDS. Some people living with HIV told me they had heard about it on radio BBC news but they could not know all the details about it. They were very happy to know all true details about it and they were committed to put my advice into action. No one of them had any opportunistic infections such as tuberculosis, pneumonia or meningitis and there was no deaths among them. This was good for them and the country of Rwanda as well as the United Nations. Finally, the mission went well and the population in the area benefited from that success. The security was assured because that population was well protected by our healthy people who even built schools in some areas. Those schools helped people who, before, had a challenge of sending their children to study far from their homes. Not only schools were built for them, but also we treated diseases of people, from the local population, who could consult our clinics, and all those services were free of charge. Local authorities and the population in the mission area were very happy about our help and they thanked us very much for it. At the end of the mission, no one of the United Nations died at my workplace and I was proud of it.

Back home in Rwanda, at the airport, I heard that I would be deployed to a hospital, which had a lot of challenges. That hospital was the MUNINI hospital and I had to wait until there was an official communication. I first went home and met with my family members: my wife and children. They were delighted to see me back home after a one-year mission in a dangerous area. My beautiful daughter called Sahaha Ariella, and who was born just days before I went to the mission, was one year old at my arrival back home from the mission area. She was healthy and I was happy to see her and the rest of my family. I had to buy a car to make transport easy for my family and I used money from the mission. The car was very nice and It could help us for different activities. For example my wife could drive it from home to the hospital without delay once a child was ill. From the mission, I had to report to Kanombe hospital where I was from and I had to work hard as usual. After some days, I had a message from the administration that the minister of health of Rwanda, Dr. Richard Sezibera, wanted me to go to his office. I went to his office and he told me that I should go to MUNINI hospital and be its medical director. I answered him that even if I had a plan to pursue my study in medicine, I could not refuse working for our country once I was asked to. I accepted and I told him that I was ready for the new deployment. After some days, I had a letter from the minister of health, officially, deploying me to MUNINI hospital as its medical director. Even if I didn't know where was located that hospital, but I was determined to go there and work very hard so that I could save human lives.

On October 17, 2010, evening, I had a phone call from human resource manager of MUNINI hospital, asking me if he would come with a driver and a pickup of the hospital the following day for my transport from Kigali to MUNINI hospital. I agreed and on October 18, 2010, around 10AM Central African Time, I met with them and we left Kigali to the southern province of Rwanda. I was curious to know such a hospital, I had heard for my first time. On the way towards the hospital, I told them to stop in Huye town and I offered them lunch as I was going to work with them for quite some time ahead. After Huye, we went to Nyaruguru district where it is located the MUNINI hospital. My impression of the area was a remote area with less development if compared to other places in Rwanda with the majority of houses built with adobe bricks and no asphalt road at its big part, then. There was no sign of high agricultural production and people were showing poverty by their physical appearance and clothes. I automatically had a feeling of doing something to contribute towards the development of the area. Finally, we arrived at the MUNINI hospital at around 5PM and I saw few buildings in a remote hospital. I visited all departments starting with the internal medicine, which was located in the nearest health center, the maternity and the pediatric department just to mention but a few. I saw few patients, who had an appearance of being poor, and old equipment. The whole hospital had about 65 old beds including twenty in the internal medicine department, twenty in the pediatric

127

department and twenty-five beds in the maternity department. There was only one operating theater room without an anesthesia machine. The hospital didn't have electricity twenty-four hours a day because it was using electricity provided by a generator for some time. There was no water and vehicles of the hospital, with jerry-cans, were daily sent to a place with a natural spring located at about 20 Kilometers or 12 Miles far from the hospital, to find the needed water. It was the most challenging hospital in the country of Rwanda, indeed. There were few patients because only ten were in the internal medicine department, fifteen in the maternity department and five patients in the pediatric department. The total, of all patients in the MUNINI hospital at that time on my arrival, was thirty. I understood that the bed occupancy rate was still low and I was decided to find its root cause, therefore to increase that occupancy rate. I already had a feeling of being committed to contribute towards the development of the MUNINI hospital and the whole area.

On October 19, 2010, I officially started to work as medical director of MUNINI hospital after a handover ceremony where were present officials from the district, the chairperson of the board of directors, the acting medical director and hospital staff. Then, the takeover event followed with signatures and speeches. I was determined to make a positive change in service delivery, training staff and infrastructure as well as equipment. The following day, I went to the first staff meeting where all health professionals including doctors, nurses and technicians were present and I explained to them my vision that was to improve service delivery in order to save human lives. I told them that the only secret for success are hardworking attitude, quick and appropriate service delivery as well as customer care. Customer care is to look after customers so that they have satisfaction with business and its services. I gave them some examples of customer care including to welcome customers, politely ask them their needs, friendly answer them and warmly explain them on each and every thing to be done for them. The mentioned attitude could give satisfaction to patients who would have an easy and quick improvement of their clinical status. I told them that it had been proven that only drugs and medical acts were not enough to treat a patient, on the other hand a good and friendly attitude was very key to ensure an uncomplicated recovery to the patient. Furthermore, I told them that when patients would be satisfied they would come back when necessary without hesitation and this behavior would have two positive impacts. First and foremost, patients would not stay at home when they would be sick. Diseases would be treated as much earlier as possible and the success in the disease treatment would be high. Finally, morbidity or the rate of disease in a population and mortality or death on large scale, would decrease. I told them that due to the poverty in the population, much people could have stayed at home and some could have consulted traditional healers but their satisfaction at hospital would bring them to consult our health professionals. Secondly, they would pay the hospital and the income would increase and allowed us to solve some problems of drug and medical equipment purchase as well as infrastructure issue. Hospital staff knew how the hospital had many challenges of not having enough drugs and frequent stock-out of some essential drugs such as antibiotics for example augmentin, cefotaxim to name but a few. Those antibiotics are normally very important to treat some infections caused by germs that are resistant to common antibiotics. For example there are some infections in ear, nose and trachea (ENT) caused by germs that are resistant to amoxicillin, a common antibiotic, which normally treats infections in ENT. When that antibiotic fails, augmentin is the next antibiotic to be given to the patient and it has been observed that augmentin has efficacy in ENT infections where amoxicillin fails. I remember a hospital staff who had a chronic tonsillitis, which is inflammation of tonsils and it is characterized by sore throat meaning pain in the throat, enlargement of tonsils, fever, trouble swallowing and large lymph nodes around the neck. It can be caused by a virus or bacterium and the most common bacterium in tonsillitis is group A β-hemolytic streptococcus. The staff was a wife with six children and she had given birth to all those children in a very short time with an interval, between them, which was less than one year. She was always operated during the process of delivering each and every child. She was a hardworking woman and she had a lot of work to do as head of department. She was weak and her weakness status was the cause of her repetitive tonsillitis. In her medical history, she mentioned she used to be treated by amoxicillin without any improvement. A blood sample was sent to the laboratory for a full blood count and the results showed that she had a bacterial infection. I gave her augmentin for seven days, after that time she was cured and since then she has not had any tonsillitis. The challenge was the price of that drug because it was expensive if compared to amoxicillin and there was a stock-out in public pharmacies. It became very difficult to buy augmentin in private pharmacies. Another example of a drug that has shown efficacy in some bacterial infections such as pneumonia, urinary tract infection, meningitis and so on and so forth is cefotaxime. It is administered by injection into a vein or muscle. Many children, with complicated pneumonia and failure of common antibiotics such as amoxicillin, have been treated by cefotaxime. The hospital had to buy it from private pharmacies when there was a need of it and it was more expensive than amoxicillin, too. With increasing patients who consulted and paid the hospital, the problem of financial resource was solved with time.

Hospital staff understood the importance of customer care and good service delivery and they were committed to make a positive change in the way they were welcoming, explaining and treating patients.

I myself was committed to motivate hospital staff so that we, all together, could reach our goals. I could focus on hearing them and solving their problems without any delays. Normally, at a health facility for example a hospital, it is always important to avoid that an employee overworks while, in the same department, others don't. Therefore, I had to put on place some organized timetables in different departments and decentralized leadership from the hospital level to the heads of those departments. I told staff that they would do daily meetings and their heads would send the report to the hospital level. I had to receive many problems and solve them without delay. An example of a problem that has been solved is on the organization of doctors. In the past, there was one doctor on call and when there was much work, he was not able to perform well and there were some delays. I decided that all doctors, in working days, could help in case there was a necessity of working in a different department and two had to be in the hospital during weekend in order to manage appropriately all cases. There was a house for doctors in the hospital and I asked them to tell me their needs to meet the new duties aimed at offering a good service delivery to patients. They listed their needs including refurbishment of the house and support in terms of getting coffee during their night work. I responded positively to their needs and all doctors were happy. They started to work very hard and there was an improvement of service delivery after telling them to change how they were working for the patients. They treated appropriately all our patients and without delay. When I arrived, doctors were four and with the new organization they could work easily without being very tired as they were complementary. Furthermore, they could share their experiences as they were complementary, which brought to each and everyone to learn more from others. On the other hand, I had to do at least one round and sometimes two rounds a day in the whole hospital including all wards where I could see patients and see their clinical status, hear them or their caregivers. I could decide on what could be done to save lives. I would always remember one time, whereby a pregnant woman had convulsion. The convulsion is violent, irregular movement of body, caused by involuntary contractions of muscles. The doctor on call thought of epilepsy. I asked him the blood pressure of the patient and her pregnancy age. The doctor told me the pregnant woman had a high blood pressure with a 37-week pregnancy. I concluded that the woman had eclampsia and I told the doctor and nurses to give her magnesium sulfate and hypertensive medication such as hydralazine. I told them to make the operating theatre room ready for an urgent caesarian section and to send blood sample for creatinine test and urine sample for proteins test, to the laboratory. Apart from a perfusion she had already had, an urine catheter was placed into the bladder of the pregnant woman through her urethra to collect urine. When the operating room was ready, I myself went to do the caesarean section with the doctor, anesthetist and two nurses. I put on sterile clothes or scrubs, bonnet, mask and apron for the theatre. I went to wash my hands and went in the operating room. The general anesthesia was given to the pregnant woman. I put on sterilized cloth or surgical gown, wash my hands with alcohol, put on sterile gloves and cleaned her abdomen with an appropriate antiseptic. I used sterile drapes to isolate where I would do an incision in her abdomen. I did an incision in her lower part of the abdomen. After doing an incision on her abdomen, I did an incision on her uterus and I performed a baby delivery without any problems. After the successful baby delivery, I sutured the uterus and the abdomen. I told the doctor to continue the treatment of magnesium sulfate and hypertensive medication while monitoring her vital signs every thirty minutes. The results from the laboratory showed the patient had proteins in urine and increased level of creatinine in her blood. The conclusion was eclampsia as final diagnosis of the patient. Fortunately, she had a good evolution and her baby was normal. Nurses and other health professionals were very motivated and they started to work very hard, too. At the end, patients were well and quickly treated and they were very happy. Their number in consultation started to grow up and even in the admission, the hospital had more patients than in the past. We did a patient satisfaction survey that showed that patients were happy. I decided to pay on time all staff of the hospital and everyone could get her or his salary at the end of each month contrary to what happened before because they used to get their monthly salaries in the following months. Furthermore, I increased their bonuses called performance based financing based on the income of the hospital and their performances. The salary and the bonus called performance based financing, were given at the same time at the end of the month before the beginning of the following month. I told all staff that I would award the best performer employee of the year. The award would be about US$118 equivalent to 100,000Rwf then, a certificate of recognition and a photo of the best performer employee at a place near the door of the morning staff hall for one year. I set up a committee in charge of election and that committee was chaired by the clinical director and the secretary was the head of nurses and midwives. Other members of the committee were all heads of departments and one representative of nurses to witness that elections were free and fair. Eligibility was for all hospital staff who worked at hospital during the ending year apart from leaders in the management committee. Members of that management committee were: the director, administrator, clinical director, human resource manager and head of nurses and midwives. Criteria to be based on during short-listing and election were: punctuality meaning being on time with regard working time including morning staff meeting, hardworking and outstanding customer care and service delivery, sacrifice, creativity, contribution towards clear one's department achievement in different evaluations and social relationship as well as professional cooperation with colleagues. At the end of the year, I had to do a party of all staff of the hospital and the event was well organized at each end of the year. Authorities of the district, members of the hospital board of directors and opinion leaders of the district as well as former employees of the hospital were invited to the party. We had a diner together and speeches followed whereby the mayor started, the head of board of directors followed and I as the director of the hospital presented to them our achievements during the completed year and targets for the coming year. I ended my speech by wishing them a happy and prosperous new year. Before going back to my seat, I finally told them that one staff had been elected by other colleagues to be the best performer employee of the completed year. I called him or her, congratulated him or her and I gave him or her a check of about U$118 and a certificate of recognition. I showed to all who were present at the party his or her photo, which would be at a place near the door of the morning meeting hall for the full next year. Normally the elected staff was excited and thanked his or her colleagues for having elected him or her and hospital leadership for having awarded him or her. He or She was determined to continue working well for the improvement of the service delivery and customer care as I had already requested it to them. I told the rest of hospital staff to follow his or her good example and even doing more than he or she did, so that another staff could be awarded the following year. This event motivated staff, too and they were ending a year with new commitments. I remember that the first elected employee was a gentleman in charge of customer care, the second was a hardworking doctor and the third was a nurse who was head of other nurses in pediatric department. What surprised me was a gift staff always gave me for what they called their grateful appreciation for my outstanding service and leadership. I told them I was surprised for the gift because I had not imagined it and I assured them I would do more for them and the patients as I had ambition to save human lives. Authorities, members of the board of directors and staff appreciated the event and they were ready to work towards a better service delivery and customer care. It was the first time that a public institution in Rwanda awarded the best performer employee of the year and later all public institutions in the country started to award that employee on labor day. Finally, they were committed to contribute so that more lives were saved for the following year.

Furthermore, I requested all hospital staff to support a fund for indigents whereby I had to pay 1% of my monthly salary and they accepted and were ready to pay 1% of their monthly salary, too. Those funds helped us to buy food, soap and community based health insurance (CBHI) for indigent people. Later on labor Day, I created another fund called "IGIHANGO" or Blood Pact as an agreement between hospital staff and we would help each other as if we had shared our blood. I was inspired by the blood pact in ancient Rwanda whereby Rwandans drank blood of each other as agreement between two people and it meant that no one among them would betray another and they were becoming as relatives. Concretely, we, at the hospital, were decided to pay about US$1.2 per person, each month for the fund. Those funds helped any staff who lost a member of his or her family just as an example of what funds helped staff for. Another example of staff who were helped by money from that fund were those who had a serious and urgent family problems such as lack of school fees for their children at the beginning of the academic year. I remember that a nutritionist of the hospital, who had children in a high school, very quickly when he brought his request to the hospital leadership, he got money from the fund to pay for their schools while he could not find such an amount from his bank in such a helpful time. Employees appreciated the essence of the fund, which motivated them, too. I told hospital staff in a morning meeting that we were in a family at MUNINI hospital and we would work not only in a team work but also in a family work. I explained the family work as work done in a family and characterized by being complementary, sharing experience and knowledge, working without having an eye of a supervisor on him or her, taking work as own business, working very hard, sacrifice and helping each other. All hospital staff appreciated the idea and they were committed to embrace it. I told an anesthetist, who had advanced knowledge in WhatsApp to be an administrator of WhatsApp group of all staff. That WhatsApp group was entitled MUNINI FAMILY and enabled us to chat, share information and experience in a family.

I could find some partners from the United States of America such as Hickey Family Foundation, through Africa Health New Horizons (AHNH), and International

Medical Corps (IMC). The Hickey Family Foundation gave funds to build a second theatre operating room, laundry, provide urgent needed equipment and train staff. I worked with AHNH and IMC in building a big and nice second theatre operating room. The hospital had only one operating room and it was a challenge when 2 patients had to be operated urgently at the same time. Furthermore, it was a big problem when we had to disinfect and sterilize the only one existing operating theatre room because it took some time while any time a patient who needed to be operated could arrive at the hospital. With the second operating room all those problems were solved and hospital staff appreciated it. Another infrastructure that helped the hospital was a laundry and for the first time, the MUNINI hospital had an appropriate place where clothes especially those from the operating theatre room were washed adequately. Before such a laundry, cleaners didn't have an appropriate place to wash clothes and equipment, and there was a high risk of infection at the hospital. The laundry put an end to that risk and that laundry eased the work of the staff. I could hear any staff of the hospital at any time and explain him or her what can be done for his or her problem at a precise time. Once I had the possibility to solve his or her problem, I did it without any delay. I remember a staff who had a problem and who requested me to allow him to go for a mission in the United Nations as a driver. He was one of the hospital drivers and he had some financial problems at home including lack of a house because he used to rent one for his family at that time. He had a family to care of and his monthly take home, which included a monthly salary and a bonus called performance based financing, was about US$105 or 90,000Rwf with US$81 or 68,658Rwf as monthly salary and US$24 or 20,894Rwf as monthly bonus. That amount of money was not enough for him who had a family with a house to be paid every month for its rent. I told him that I was supportive of him so that he would go to the United Nations mission and find some money for a house. Furthermore, I gave him hope that as he was going to that mission officially, I would hire another driver temporarily and when he came back, his job would still be there for him. He was very happy because I answered him positively and he thanked me so much. I remember that I hired another driver to replace him temporarily at his departure. When he came back from the mission, I told him that he was going to be in his job as I had promised it to him. Later, he told me that he was successful in building his own house and I was happy about it. I encouraged him by telling him to work very hard and reach more goals. As I was head of the board of directors of the district pharmacy, when it was needed to hire a driver for a new vehicle at that pharmacy, I informed the one who had been hired temporarily at the hospital and he could succeed to get a job, too. He appreciated what I did for him and he was decided to work very hard, too, in his new job.

In terms of motivating staff who were members of management committee, I had to take them to a retreat far from the hospital where we could even do a good planning of hospital activities. Those members of the management committee appreciated such a retreat and they were committed to contribute in order to achieve our goal.

Moreover, due to few staff at the hospital including only 4 doctors for the hospital in a district of 300,000 people according to Rwanda population census 2012, 14 sectors and 16 health centers, I could not request any leave not to worsen the gap of doctors.

In an evaluation done by the ministry of health, we could be the best in the whole country with 96.4% in total, including 100% in customer care.

I remember that patients increased 5 times in 4 years with our improved service delivery and customer care, from 1892 in 2008 to 10370 in 2012.

The bed occupancy rate doubled in 4 years from 41% in 2008 to 82% in 2012.

The MUNINI hospital had those achievements due to motivation of staff but that hospital had many challenges. Those challenges were: to be the only hospital in the whole district of NYARUGURU. This district had, as above mentioned, 300,000 people according to Rwanda Population Census, 2012, on surface area of 1,010 Km^2 with roads in bad condition, 14 sectors and 16 health centers such as: COKO, KIBEHO, NYAMYUMBA, MUGANZA, NYABIMATA, KIVU, RUHERU, RUNYOMBYI, MUGANZA, CYAHINDA, MARABA, NGOMA, KABILIZI and MUNINI. All those health centers were transferring to MUNINI hospital, which had only 65 beds and 4 ambulances but only one ambulance was in good condition. The district, where is located the hospital, is one of eight districts of the southern province of Rwanda. Those districts of the southern province included NYAMAGABE, HUYE, GISAGARA, NYANZA, RUHANGO, MUHANGA, KAMONYI and NYARUGURU. It took about 1 hour and a half to transfer patients from the MUNINI hospital to the nearest referral hospital called BUTARE University Teaching hospital. The MUNINI hospital was working in rehabilitated houses that were belonging to an agricultural project called DANK or Agricultural Development of NSHILI-KIVU or "DEVELOPPEMENT AGRICOLE NSHILI-KIVU" in French. The infrastructure were not appropriate and they were not enough. There were no surgery, intensive care and ophthalmology departments just to mention but a few. Many departments of the MUNINI hospital were located in the nearest health center including internal medicine, radiography, human resource, accounting, mortuary and supervision departments. The hospital had not enough equipment. It didn't have a functional anesthesia machine, equipment for emergency cases, monitoring machine in maternity department, resuscitation trolley in pediatric department, an autoclave for sterilization and enough incubators because there were only 2 while at least 4 were needed. There was no appropriate generator because the one at the hospital had only 6 kilovolt-ampere (KVA) while it was needed a more powerful one of 50KVA. Sometimes, when the 6-KVA generator was not in function because it could not work for the whole night, we used candles in the hospital. There was no software in accounting department and it took much time and work to make a financial report than when there could have been such a software in the hospital. There was lack of enough personnel because when I arrived at the MUNINI hospital in October, 2010, there were only 63 staff while the minimum should be at least 83. There was lack of enough training in staff and for example only 2 nurses out of 12 in maternity were trained in emergency, obstetric and neonatal care (EMONC). There were diseases in the whole district and there were the top 5 that included: respiratory tract infection, which represented 37.7% of all cases in 2012; intestinal worms representing 13.8%; gastritis 9.8%; trauma 8.8% and dental infection 6.6% according to health management information system (HMIS) of 2012. In October, 2010, at my arrival at MUNINI hospital, there were no water and electricity.

I had to think several times what I would do to overcome those challenges. I was decided not to give up. Sometimes, I had solutions to some problems late at night while sleeping, and I could have in my mind an idea at around 3AM. On the other hand, I had a feeling that "there is no single problem that can be solved by losing control". Apart from being a hospital of many challenges, the MUNINI hospital was in a remote area, and I could not find areas for entertainment after work. I avoided drinking alcohol and I could stay at the hospital 24 hours, 5 days a week (24/5). In the weekend, I could make sure that a team of doctors, nurses and other health professionals were ready on call at the hospital and go to see my family in Kigali. The team on call could phone me if there was a problem they could not solve themselves. I remember a patient who had a cranial trauma in a road accident and the doctor on call, phoned me to ask me advice on an antibiotic to give that patient who had a good Glasgow Coma Scale of 14/15. The Glasgow Coma Scale (GCS) is an assessment done on a traumatic head injury patient in order to know the level of consciousness of the patient and the severity of the injury. The GCS has 3 elements including: eye; motor and verbal. With regard eye, when the patient does not open eyes, we give 1; when eyes are opened in response to pain, we give

2; when he or she opens eyes in response to voice, we give 3; when the patient opens eyes spontaneously, we give 4. On motor point of view: when the patient does not do any movements, we give 1; when the patient does extension to a painful stimuli, we give 2; when he or she does abnormal flexion to a painful stimuli, we give 3; when the patient does flexion and withdraw to a painful stimuli, we give 4; when he or she localizes a painful stimuli, we give 5 and when the patient obeys command, we give 6. On verbal scale: when the patient makes no sound, we give 1; when he or she makes sounds, we give 2; when the patient pronounces some words, we give 3; when he or she is confused or disoriented, we give 4 and when the patient is oriented and speaks normally, we give 5. When GCS is < 8-9, the brain injury is severe; when it is between 9 and 12, the brain injury is moderate and when GCS is ≥ 13, the brain injury is minor. The maximum Glasgow Coma Scale is 15 and the patient had a minor head injury because he had 14/15. I told him to give the patient ceftriaxone, which is normally good for such a cranial trauma case because it is a broad-spectrum antibiotic. The patient had a good evolution and on X-ray he had not any fracture of cranial bones. Another example of a doctor who called when he was on call while I was in a weekend in my family is on child who had an infection after circumcision. The child got an antibiotic called amoxicillin without success. His parents brought him to the hospital. They called me and asked me advice on antibiotic to give him. I told the parents to send to me the picture that described the wound and that wound was yellow due to infection. I told the doctor that he should give him augmentin. After five days, the infection was treated and the child had no longer the disease.

When back to the hospital, I could write, a plan of activities that I would do the whole week, in my diary. Among activities, I had to write clinical activities including solutions to existing problems. The worst problem, which was at the MUNINI hospital when I arrived at that hospital in 2010, was a high neonatal death rate of 77/1000. Neonatal death rate is a number of deaths during the first 28 completed days of life per 1000 live births in a given year or period. I first made an analysis of causes and I found that main causes were staff who were not focused sufficiently on their job, delay transfer from health centers and lack of electricity and water at the hospital level. Staff were not focused sufficiently on their job because they were taking vital signs of new born babies at irregular time and they could not act on time to save lives. Furthermore, there was no proper department of neonatology and one staff could come from another department such as internal medicine and enter in the new born place without any measures of hygiene. Therefore, there were many infections to new born babies and those infections were one of the causes of their deaths. On the other hand, there was a delay in transferring new born babies from health centers, which were in the MUNINI hospital catchment area and new born babies could arrive almost dead at the hospital. Staff who received those babies could not do anything that could make them alive. Furthermore, there were some places that could not have a health center to facilitate people to reach it. At the hospital, there were no electricity, water and there were insufficient incubators, because there were 2 instead of being at least 4, those incubators could not be functional 24 hours in 7 days. When the 6 KVA generator, of the hospital, was off, as it could not work the whole day, a new born baby in an incubator could die due to hypothermia. Main causes of new born babies at the hospital were: hypothermia, prematurity and infection.

I had to take some measures to solve the above mentioned problems.

On the staff not sufficiently focused on their job, I was decided to explain the hospital staff in each and every morning staff meeting the importance of making a regular and thorough follow-up of a new born baby. Furthermore, I was decided to lead by example and I myself had to make a follow-up of all new born babies by making a quick ward round at least twice a day where those babies were hospitalized with their mothers in the maternity department. Every time, I had to check their vital signs especially their temperature, respiratory and cardiac rates as well as oxygen saturation. I also had to check if the treatment prescribed by a doctor on duty was correct and if it was given to the new born baby correctly. When there was a mistake, I had to call the doctor, advise him and we could correct the treatment. Doctors and nurses started to work very hard and be more focused on their work in general and the health of the new born babies in particular. Furthermore, I had an idea of finding a small room, which could be available all the time and be used as a neonatology department. I requested one room to the nurses who had two rooms that they used for their rest in the maternity department and they gave me the room where I put four beds for the new neonatology department.

On the other hand, I remembered that I had studied, in the faculty of medicine, "Kangaroo" method that was about a mother to put a premature baby on her chest and cover the baby to increase the temperature of the premature baby from hypothermia to normal temperature. At the MUNINI hospital, every premature baby was condemned to death because of hypothermia, as there were no electricity and incubators that could function 24 hours and seven days. But with the use of "Kangaroo" method, premature babies were no longer condemned to death, because that method helped us to raise their temperature from low to normal temperature.

On another issue that was causing neonatal deaths, the delayed transfer system, I realized that MUNINI hospital had fifteen health centers then and sometimes it took a lot of time for an ambulance to leave the hospital then go to a health center and come back to the hospital with a patient. This transfer process took about two hours or more and this process was actually among main causes of neonatal deaths because a new born baby with respiratory distress could not survive without a treatment normally provided at the hospital level. After two months, there have been sixteen health centers in the whole district or the MUNINI hospital catchment area. I decided to decentralize ambulances from the hospital to the health centers and two ambulances were kept at the hospital while two were at the health center level. In each and every corner of the district, we had an ambulance that shortened the transfer process and consequently, deaths decreased. For example, five health centers such as MARABA, CYAHINDA, NYANTANGA and NGOMA as well as NGERA shared one ambulance, which had been at the MUNINI hospital before. The ambulance was positioned at MARABA health center, which was in the center of all five health centers. Transfers from all those five health centers to MUNINI hospital was done very quickly because the ambulance was near those health centers. On the other hand, all five health centers had to contribute for the fuel and maintenance of the ambulance because the management, of the ambulance, belonged to the five health centers.

A second decentralized ambulance from the hospital, was shared with two health centers in deep remote area and it was positioned at RUHERU health center. Those health centers were RUHERU and RUNYOMBYI. Some patients could wait more than two hours to reach MUNINI hospital from their health centers because of bad roads and the distance between them and the hospital. The distance between RUHERU health center and the hospital was about forty kilometers or twenty-five miles. I remember a new ambulance that had a broken chassis from the hospital to RUHERU health center while it was sent to RUHERU health center to bring a patient to MUNINI hospital and it was due to very bad road in that area. We informed the ministry of health and we sent the ambulance, which had the broken chassis, to the headquarters of the ministry of health in the capital city of Rwanda, Kigali. The ministry of health sent a message to the manufacturers, informing them about the broken chassis of their new ambulance without any accidents. The manufacturers from South Africa, could not understand what happened to their vehicle and they planned a visit aimed at understanding the causes of such a broken chassis of a new vehicle without an accident. When they arrived at the MUNINI hospital, they went with a hospital driver to see the road between the MUNINI hospital and RUHERU health center where the vehicle had the above mentioned problem. When they saw how bad was that road, they didn't arrive at the health center and they came back to the hospital saying that the very bad status of the road could have been the cause of the broken chassis. But as we had later decentralized an ambulance based at RUHERU health center for that health center and RUNYOMBYI health center, transfers from both health centers did not delay anymore and deaths including neonatal deaths decreased significantly.

A third ambulance was given by Pope John Paul the second to KIBEHO health center, which was belonging to the Roman catholic church. That health center was helped by the government of Rwanda, which especially provided salaries of staff. I had to convince the head of the health center who was a roman catholic sister so that the new ambulance would be shared by KIBEHO, NYAMYUMBA and KABILIZI health centers to solve a problem of delay in transfer process. I promised her that I would convince the heads of the other two health centers to contribute for maintenance and fuel of the new ambulance. All the heads of the three health centers accepted to contribute to the management of new ambulance by paying for its fuel and maintenance. People in that area were very happy and they could have an ambulance near them and when needed without any delay. Deaths including neonatal deaths started to decrease in that area and it was a success for our health system.

Furthermore, another problem that I had to work on when I arrived at the MUNINI hospital, was the lack of a health center in one of the areas of its catchment area and that area was called NGERA. The population of the NGERA sector had to go to another district of Rwanda called HUYE for their treatment and it was a very challenging situation for the whole population in that area. The distance from NGERA health center to a neighboring health facility was very long and it took about one hour to reach that neighboring health center. This great distance discouraged many people who could not find where to be treated near them. Some people preferred not to consult on one hand due to that great distance and on the other hand because of poverty, others could go to traditional healers. Even those traditional healers could not have enough capacity to do a diagnosis of a disease because they were not performing a simple test for malaria. A patient could die because of malaria while in another sector of the district, there was a health center with a laboratory to perform blood smear for malaria and availability of anti malaria drugs like Coartem and Quinine. The majority of patients who had malaria, in a sector where there was a health center, were treated without any problems. There was also a high risk of having a complicated case because of delay in consulting a health professional and treatment of such a case could be challenging with a high risk of failing in its management. There were many deaths including neonatal deaths due to lack of a health center. I had to make a decision to contribute towards its beginning because they already had houses but without equipment and staff. I organized a meeting with all health centers and I explained all heads of health centers that we could contribute and help NGERA health center start working. They accepted and the MUNINI hospital started by contributing in terms of personnel by paying two A2 nurses every month, providing some medical equipment of maternity department, laboratory and office such as tables and chairs. The hospital of MUNINI also provided a vehicle for transport of all equipment offered to NGERA health center. On January 3, 2011, I went to the ceremony of the inauguration of NGERA health center. It was wonderful and helpful to the population of NGERA sector because they had a new health center, ever, near them. People started to consult on time, they were treated appropriately and transferred on time, which decreased deaths including neonatal deaths.

On the other hand, I could advocate for electricity and the hospital of MUNINI had it, which helped so much in terms of saving lives especially new born babies. We could treat patients anytime including pregnant women who had to be operated for a caesarean section. We could not delay in using an operating theatre room because it had permanent electricity and we could therefore avoid many deaths of new born babies with our rapidity in operating pregnant women who had indications for a c-section. I had to advocate the water supply and Family Health International (FHI 360) a non-governmental organization from the United States of America offered the hospital of MUNINI about twenty-four thousand US dollars equivalent to twenty million Rwandan francs, which allowed our hospital to get water. That water contributed to decrease infections in the hospital particularly in the operating room and therefore saved many lives including new born babies' lives. I could contact Global Fund and it provided two incubators to the hospital of MUNINI. The total number of those incubators became four, which was the required number of incubators at the MUNINI hospital. I could get another room, which was used for used clothes from the operating room, and I used it for the four incubators.

All those factors contributed to decrease neonatal death rate from 77/1000 in 2010 according to health management information system 2010 (HMIS 2010) to 2/1000 in 2015 according to health management information system 2015 (HMIS 2015). It was amazing and MUNINI hospital, which could have been closed due to bad performance, became the success story in the ministry of health particularly and in Rwanda generally.

The prime minister of Rwanda declared in a 2012 meeting of all directors of hospitals in Rwanda, that I was the best director of hospital in the country for the year 2011 and the MUNINI hospital was the best hospital in terms of service delivery for that year and countrywide.

At my arrival at MUNINI hospital in 2010, there were many deaths of pregnant women and I remember that four mothers died in that year. As all staff should be involved, even hospital supervisors of health centers, had to do supervision in the hospital and each department in the hospital had a supervisor who was responsible of. Among those supervisors, there was one who had been head of all nurses in maternity department, and she was appointed to be the supervisor of the maternity department and she actually helped staff in that department. Later at MUNINI hospital, started an amazing system called rapid SMS that was aiming at receiving telephone messages sent from the community and health center alerting staff on ambulance at hospital on maternal emergency cases such as bleeding on pregnancy or convulsion on pregnancy and so on and so forth. I remember that many pregnant women who had bleeding could be saved without any delay due to such a wonderful system. Community health workers who were in charge of pregnant women in a village had to make a follow-up on regular basis and they had a telephone so that when a problem occurred to any of those pregnant women in a village, the community health worker was the first to send an alerting message with an immediate response from the hospital. I could monitor each and every community health worker based on the system. For example a community health worker who was active, could send updating messages on pregnant women in a village while the one who was not active could not. The system could show the percentage of active community health workers in a health center catchment area and those who were not. In a morning staff meeting, I had to get a presentation on rapid SMS from a staff of the hospital. Health centers that didn't have 100% active community health workers were called and requested them to tell all community health workers, in their catchment areas, to be active and the following day there was an improvement. The rapid SMS system could show a pregnant woman who had reach the time to deliver and I could tell an employee to call and tell the community health worker who was in charge of that woman to bring her to the hospital for examination and good management of that pregnancy. There was a say, particularly at MUNINI hospital, that "No more preventable deaths should occur" and everything was done so that preventable deaths didn't occur.

With my efforts, to decrease deaths in general including deaths of pregnant women, and collaboration with all hospital staff, those maternal deaths were decreased from 4 in 2010 according to health management information system (HMIS 2010) to 0 in 2011 according to health management information system (HMIS 2011). It was incredible and I would never forget such a great achievement.

On the other hand, there were many cases of malaria in 2010 because all confirmed malaria cases were 11983. I was decided to work with supervisors including community health supervisor, health centers and community health workers and a sensitization was done based on explaining the population how to do prevention from getting malaria. The preventive measures were basically sleeping in an insecticide treated net. At the beginning all people didn't sleep in those nets because some said they were increasing their body temperature and they could be very hot, others said they were allergic to those insecticide treated nets. In sensitization, they could understand that the worst thing was to get malaria, which could kill a person while all those other feelings or uncomforting behaviors could not. The insecticide treated nets were distributed to those who didn't have any and the distribution was based on member of family numbers so that all people sleeping on each bed in a family had a net. For example, parents had their own insecticide treated net and children sleeping on a bed had to get their own net. Confirmed malaria cases decreased from 11983 in 2010 according to health management information system 2010 (HMIS 2010) to 2886 in 2012 according to health management information system 2012 (HMIS 2012).

There has been an outbreak of measles in the catchment area of MUNINI hospital at Burundi-Rwanda border. It was in 2010, when many children had measles in at least three sector of the district of NYARUGURU. Those three sectors were: RUHERU, BUSANZE and NYABIMATA, all located at the border of Rwanda and Burundi. RUHERU sector is located in south of the district and it had about 37,328 population (2015). The first case of measles appeared in that sector and a child had fever, cough, red eyes, muscle ache or pain, runny nose, sore throat or pain in the throat, light sensitivity, white spots inside the mouth called Koplik spots and widespread skin rash. I concluded that it was a case of measles and I requested blood sample for confirmation. The sample was sent to the national referral laboratory to test it and tell us whether there was a virus of measles in. Measles is normally caused by a virus called paramyxovirus and it is highly contagious because it is transmitted in tiny droplets when a patient infected coughs, breathes and sneezes. We could give the patient antipyretic and pain killer to decrease the temperature and pain of that child, humidifier to treat cough, fluids to avoid dehydration and vitamin A that normally helps a patient to fight against measles. The patient improved well and the result came confirming that it was a case of measles. On the other hand, there were other similar cases in RUHERU, BUSANZE in south of the district with a population of about 28,511 (2015) and NYABIMATA in south-west of the district with a population of 17,777 (2015). I myself decided to drive a pickup from the hospital to the centre of immunization located in Kigali. As I had already talked with authorities in the ministry of health and Rwanda biomedical center, I had vaccines to vaccinate the three sectors. The following day the localized vaccination campaign started and it was successfully ended with all children, who had to get the vaccine, were vaccinated.

The 2010 measles outbreak at Burundi-Rwanda border was quickly stopped without a single death. This was an achievement and I was proud of it.

With regard immunization in general, MUNINI hospital had a good performance and in June 2015, the immunization rate of most of vaccines was 100% in the catchment area of the hospital. Factors of such a huge success were working with community health workers, sensitization of population and outreach strategies as well as meetings with heads of health centers. Community health workers were trained and briefed and tasked to sensitize population on importance of immunization. Some people had bad behavior and said that some vaccines were bad for their children who could be sterile due to those vaccines according to their believes. But with community health workers who could reach each and every family, sensitized all people based on what they had been told in different meetings and training and the population could understand the importance of vaccines. On the other hand, there were outreach strategies at health center level whereby health professionals didn't wait people to bring their children to the health center. They had to go to a place that was near targeted people who were in need of immunization and such a strategy increased numbers of vaccinated children. Finally, in a coordination meeting that was organized by the hospital, health center representatives were participants including head of each health center in the hospital catchment area, hospital representatives, district health representatives and it was chaired by the director of hospital. Data were presented, including those relating to immunization, and health centers that had performed well were congratulated and they were told to tell their success story to others specifically factors of good performance. Health centers that had bad performance were asked to explain the reasons of their bad performance. Solutions to the problems that had caused it, were highlighted and they were requested to implement those solutions without delay and a follow-up was done. For Human Papillomavirus (HPV) vaccine, there was a vaccination rate of 100% in MUNINI hospital catchment area. HPV is a type of virus that can cause abnormal growth of soft tissue from warts to cervical cancer. HPV has more than 100 subtypes, 40 of which can pass through sexual contact. HPV passes between people through skin-to-skin contact and it can be transmitted from a mother to her baby during birth. There are some risk factors to contract HPV. Those risk factors are: having a high number of intimate partners; sex with someone who has had several intimate partners; a weakened immune system, for example, due to HIV; areas of damaged skin, personal contact with surfaces, for example, warts, where HPV exposure has occurred; cigarette smoking is a risk factor for cervical cancer and among HPV-infected women, current and former smokers have roughly two to three times the incidence of invasive cancer; birth control pills or oral contraceptives are a risk factor for cervical cancer and long-term use of oral contraceptives is associated with increased risk of cervical cancer. Women who have used oral contraceptives for 5 to 9 years have about three times the incidence of invasive cancer. HPV may not cause symptoms at once, but they can appear years later as warts, especially genital warts or cancer, particularly cervical cancer. Genital warts may appear as a small bump, cluster of bumps, or stem-like protrusions. They commonly affect the vulva in women, or possibly the cervix, and the penis or scrotum in men. They may also appear around the anus and in the groin, which is the area between the lower abdomen and the thigh on either side of the body. The uterine cervix is the lowest portion of a woman's connecting the uterus and the vagina. HPV 16 and 18, result in around 70% of cervical cancer cases. Women with early cervical cancer and pre-cancers usually have no symptoms. Symptoms often do not begin until cancer becomes invasive and grows into nearby tissue. When this happens the most important symptoms are: abnormal vaginal bleeding, such as bleeding after vaginal sex, bleeding after menopause, bleeding and spotting between periods, and having menstrual periods that are longer or heavier than usual, bleeding after douching or after a pelvic exam may also occur; an unusual discharge from the vagina, the discharge may contain blood or may occur between periods or after your menopause; pelvic pain and pain during sex. Tests to evaluate for HPV or HPV-related cervical cellular changes include a Pap smear, a DNA test and the use of acetic acid (vinegar). A Pap smear collects cells from the surface of the cervix and may reveal any cellular abnormalities, which may lead to cancer. The DNA test will evaluate for the high-risk types of HPV. At times, a biopsy of any abnormal areas may be necessary. Some preventive measures can reduce the risk of contracting HPV and those measures are: HPV vaccination for example Gardasil that reduces the risk of cancerous and precancerous changes of the cervix and perineum by about 93% and the vaccine is between 92% and 100% effective against HPV 16 and 18. The vaccine is given between 9 and 26 years and specifically at age 11 and 12 years, to reduce the risk of contracting cervical cancer and other cancers. The vaccine is given in two doses, 6 to 12 months apart; practicing abstinence or being in a monogamous sexual relationship; not having sex while there are visible genital warts; and for more preventive measures for cervical cancer are screening by Papanicolaou test or Pap test; Nutrition and vitamin A is associated with a lower risk as are vitamin B12, vitamin C, vitamin E and beta-carotene. In the treatment of cervical cancer there are surgical intervention, radiotherapy and chemotherapy. Surgical intervention such as hysterectomy, the removal of the whole uterus including part of vagina, in microinvasive cancer, may have better outcomes than radiotherapy. Radiotherapy can be used in all cancer stages where surgical options do not exist because cervical cancers are radiosensitive. Chemotherapy has been found to be more effective than radiotherapy alone. Warts that result from HPV will often resolve without treatment. However, there are medications that can be applied to the skin to remove the warts, these include podophyllin, trichloroacetic acid. Surgical interventions may be necessary and include: electrocautery, which is an electrical current used to burn the abnormal areas; surgical removal; cryotherapy, which uses liquid nitrogen to freeze abnormal areas; laser therapy whereby a light beam removes unwanted tissue. Worldwide, cervical cancer is both the fourth-most common cause of cancer and deaths from cancer in women. In 2012, an estimated 528,000 cases of cervical cancer occurred, with 266,000 deaths. About 80% of cervical cancers occur in developing countries. It is the most frequently detected cancer during pregnancy with an occurrence of 1.5 to 12 for every 100,000 pregnancies. In 2018, there were about 570,000 new cases of cervical cancer, which caused about 311,000 deaths in the world. In Rwanda, cervical cancer incidence was 49.4/100,000 in 2012 according to World Health Organization (WHO). In HPV vaccine launching particularly, MUNINI hospital was chosen to host the official launching of that vaccine at the national level. That choice of the MUNINI hospital was a sign that the hospital was recognized for its achievements of different health activities and organization. I started working on it the day I heard that good news. I first of all informed all hospital staff and requested them to work on it, too. Secondly, I informed the district authorities who were very happy about the wonderful news. The district decided that a site where would happen such a launching and that site was the KIBEHO site where many people could gather without problem. Furthermore, the district appointed the executive secretary as the master of ceremony of the event and three nearby sectors were informed that they would sensitize their populations to participate to the event. Journalists were informed and an advertisement was sent to the national radio for the

Rwandan population and that advertisement was telling people about the importance of HPV vaccine and its official launching at MUNINI hospital. Furthermore, I had to give an interview on cervical cancer, its signs and symptoms, diagnosis, prevention based on HPV vaccine to be launched nationwide, treatment and statistics. People reacted mentioning that they were informed about that disease and interested in the vaccine that would save lives. This message was very important because many cases of cervical cancer arrived at the hospital in a very advanced cancer stage and nothing could be done to save such patients. I remember a woman who came to the hospital and she was cachectic. She had fatigue, anorexia, pallor, abnormal vaginal bleeding, and cervical edema. She had a cervical cancer in an advanced stage and on chest X-ray, she had radiologic signs of metastatic cancer in the lungs. She was in her last stage cervical cancer. We managed to give her blood and painkillers. After having stabilized her, she was transferred to Butare University Teaching hospital and after some days she was transferred back because there was no other further possible treatment. As she was still stable, she was sent back home with painkillers and she was told to come back to MUNINI hospital, once her status became worse. That is why we were committed to continue sensitizing people about the cervical cancer, consult without delay and young girls to prevent such a cancer by getting a HPV vaccine.

On its launching, there were many authorities from the government of Rwanda, representatives of Global Alliance for Vaccines and Immunization (GAVI), which is a public-private global health partnership dedicated to "immunization for all". Other representatives present, were from the district and there were many people from the nearest sectors and students from high schools in the district. The HPV vaccine was given to girl students selected for the event and followed by speeches from a minister who was representing the government of Rwanda and the mayor of the district. They were mentioning the launching of such an important vaccine and thanking partners such as GAVI for the support in that matter, UNICEF and other organizations. Journalists were present to cover the event and tell the story to the world. After the vaccination launching and speeches, followed socialization with all people present. Students and population from the nearest sectors got a soft drink and each and everyone had at least one soda, while authorities went to a catholic sisters' motel, near the launching site, for their lunch. The event was a success and I was proud of it.

On the other hand, I had a partnership with Starkey Hearing Foundation through an American global health non-governmental organization working in Rwanda. Starkey Hearing Foundation is a foundation committed to help people, with hearing problems, who can't afford the management of their diseases. That foundation accepted to come working for people who had such a hearing problem in MUNINI hospital catchment area. We sensitized all people who would need a help in that matter and I gave an interview to a journalist of a national television on the campaign. The whole country, including the district where is located the hospital, knew the event. Furthermore, that information was given to the district authorities and community health workers who would give it to the population of the district. 900 patients were expected but at the end of the 3-day campaign, there were more than nine hundred patients. I remember that on the first day, there were lines of people and I realized that the campaign was needed by the population. Not only people from the district of NYARUGURU, where the MUNINI hospital is located, but also patients from other districts of Rwanda came to seek treatment of their hearing diseases. Staff of Starkey Hearing Foundation trained and worked with the hospital staff deployed to that event. Those staff of the hospital could do a follow-up of treated patients who lived in the district. We could give hearing aids for free to all patients who were in need of them. One hearing aid had a value of about $500 equivalent to 425,000Rwf and two hearing aids had a value of $1000 or 850,000Rwf. People were very happy to get them because they could hear then. As some people still came after 3 days, 1 day was added on to the campaign and after 4 days, we had 92 more than expected with a total of 992 hearing patients successfully treated. I was proud of having contributed to that campaign that solved hearing problems of all mentioned people.

Furthermore, I could start a one stop center for Gender based violence (GBV) and that one stop center had different departments in the same building. Those departments were a consultation room of a doctor for GBV patients, laboratory, anti retroviral drugs (ARV), mental health, a room for police person as legal department representative. The building was one of many destroyed buildings in the hospital. Buildings that were belonging to an agricultural project became the MUNINI hospital in 2008 and they had been destroyed during 1994 genocide

162

against Tutsi in Rwanda. Among all those buildings, there was one that had to be rehabilitated before becoming a one stop center for GBV. I had to find funds for the rehabilitation and I could work with partners to make the center a reality. After some works, the center was launched and people were very happy because it would solve the gender violence problem among other problems. Patients could get a service delivery from different departments in the same building. A victim of GBV who had to get a consultation from a doctor, be tested in laboratory, getting drugs from ARV department, be counseled in mental health department and see a police person for legal issues, could do it in the same building. That eased the service delivery for the patient who was not obliged to go far in order to get that needed service delivery, which moreover became very quick.

Another problem was malnutrition and in Rwanda stunting was 44% in 2010 according to 2010 Rwanda Demographic Health Survey (RDHS 2010). The MUNINI hospital is in NYARUGURU district, which was one of the poorest districts in Rwanda. The district had an acidic soil in its biggest part and agricultural production was not high with one of the highest levels of malnutrition countrywide. I had to work on it by working with partners so that, first of all, a district plan to eliminate malnutrition (DPEM) existed. I had to take a team from the hospital, health centers and other partners to a retreat in the western part of Rwanda, precisely in RUSIZI district for that malnutrition elimination plan DPEM. From the hospital, were present nutritionist, supervisor in charge of community, supervisor in charge of data management, supervisor in charge of monitoring and evaluation, other supervisors, members of management committee such as medical director, clinical director, administrator, human resource manager and head nursing. From the health center, there were a nutritionist, supervisor in charge of community and head of health center. There were other partners including partners, from UNICEF and ministry of health, who joined us for that important plan aimed at eliminating malnutrition. We had to work very hard so that we had a useful plan in few days. The period of that plan to eliminate malnutrition was from 2011 to 2013. In situation analysis, the NYARUGURU district had 11.4% children who had malnutrition according to an assessment done at the national level. In 2009, the district had 2132 children who were affected by malnutrition including 584 who had severe acute malnutrition and 1548 children who had moderate acute malnutrition according to that assessment. Causes of malnutrition were:

insufficient food intake, infectious diseases, inadequate access to clean water, insufficient access to health facilities, acidic soil, and big size of families. Especially, children under 5 years were the most affected by malnutrition and malnutrition was chronic during the whole year in the district. The most affected population by malnutrition was at NYUNGWE belt in five sectors such as BUSANZE, RUHERU, NYABIMATA, MUGANZA and KIVU.

The plan had some strategies such as strengthen identification and management of under nutrition, strengthen and scale up community-based nutrition interventions/programs (CBNP) to prevent and manage malnutrition in children under 5 years and in pregnant and lactating women. Other strategies were: eliminate micronutrient deficiencies, develop a plan to eliminate malnutrition based on multi-sectors approach, prevent and manage nutritional deficiencies and excess-related diseases, behavior change communication, coordinate nutrition partners and do monitoring and evaluation of nutrition activities at all levels. There were expected results to each and every strategy. On strategy 1, strengthen identification and management of under nutrition, the expected results were: targeted groups were effectively identified, treated, followed up and integrated into community programs to ensure that malnutrition didn't occur. On strategy 2, strengthen and scale up community-based nutrition interventions/programs (CBNP) to prevent malnutrition in children under 5 years and in pregnant and lactating women, the expected results were: 100% of all villages had implemented community-led nutrition interventions within the first year of implementation of this strategy, 80% of villages had adopted optimal IYCF (Infant and Young Child Feeding) practices, nutrition of pregnant and lactating women, appropriate hygiene practices, use of LLIN (Long-Lasting Impregnated Net), family planning, HIV/AIDS prevention and community based health insurance (CBHI) called "MUTUELLE DE SANTE" and 40% of villages had integrated early childhood development (ECD), community integrated management childhood illness (C IMCI) and community-led nutrition interventions. On strategy 3, eliminate micronutrient deficiencies, the expected results were: 100% of children aged between 6 and 59 months had received micronutrient supplements according to the national protocol, 100% of women in post partum period had received a vitamin A dose after delivery, 100% of pregnant women had received iron-folic acid supplementation during antenatal care (ANC), 100% of centrally processed foods identified in national legislation had been fortified with vitamin A, iron and other micronutrients according to national standards, 100% of salt sold in Rwanda had been iodized according to national standards and 50% of children aged between 6 to 24 months had received adequate fortified food complements (sprinkles or fortified complementary foods). On strategy 4, develop a plan to eliminate malnutrition based on multi-sectors approach, the expected results were: district had developed plan to eliminate malnutrition through multi-sectors approach and district had implemented the plan to eliminate malnutrition at the community level. On strategy 5, prevent and manage nutritional deficiencies and excess-related diseases, the expected results were: 100% of households had been sensitized on the risk factors and dangers associated with overweight and poor dietary combinations. On strategy 6, behavior change communication, the expected results were: 100% of villages had received behavior change messages and district had included behavior change communication in the plan to eliminate malnutrition. On strategy 7, coordinate nutrition partners, the expected results were: partner coordination in the management of malnutrition had been strengthened and duplication of support to nutrition activities had been avoided. Finally on strategy 8, do monitoring and evaluation of nutrition activities at all levels, the expected results were: nutrition activities had been improved, monitoring and evaluation (M&E) guide for nutrition activities had been available and integrated in health management information system (HMIS) of the ministry of health and information of nutrition situation had been regularly analyzed and disseminated.

On the other hand, there were activities to be done in the plan for elimination of malnutrition. Those activities were: training of health care providers on management of acute malnutrition protocol and the target was 60 health care providers at the health center level and 664 at the village level; annual district screening and identification of malnutrition using middle upper arm circumference (MUAC) for children who had under 5 years of age, pregnant women and lactating women while the target was that all children who were under 5 years of age, all pregnant and lactating women on risk of malnutrition, were identified; and regular procurement of nutrition commodities such as F75, F100 and so on and so forth and the target was to avoid stock out of those nutrition commodities. Other activities were: conduct weekly and monthly supervisions of nutrition services from district hospital to health centers and the target was to improve the level of nutrition services; assess, according to the national protocol, the nutrition status of all children, pregnant and lactating women seeking health care at health facilities and the target was nutrition status of all children, pregnant and lactating women seeking health care at health facilities was known; assess the nutrition status of all children and pregnant and lactating women in specific departments such as tuberculosis (TB), HIV, maternal child health (MCH) and family planning (FP) departments and the target was all targeted groups were screened for malnutrition; nutrition counseling (including peer learning) sessions and the target was all pregnant women received nutrition counseling; and iron, folic acid and vitamin B supplementation during antenatal care (ANC) visits and the target was all pregnant women received iron and folic acid supplementation during ANC visits. There were many more activities in the plan, including: distribution of community health worker (CHW) community-based nutrition programs (CBNP) booklets; sensitization of local leaders on CBNP; organization of training sessions for service providers on CBNP and organization of community kitchen at village level. There were in the plan to eliminate malnutrition: nutrition counseling and promotion sessions on infant and young child feeding (IYCF), nutrition of pregnant and lactating women, nutrition care and support for people living with HIV as well as appropriate hygiene practices; sensitization of the community based on findings from the situation analysis; organization of community participatory planning of multisectoral interventions; promotion and protection of optimal IYCF practices including infected and/or affected by HIV/AIDS. There were activities such as: early initiation of breastfeeding within 1 hour after birth; exclusive breastfeeding for 6 months; appropriate complementary feeding, breastfeeding then complement, up to 2 years; peer learning, counseling, sessions on optimal IYCF practices; training of health workers on code implementation and monitoring, promotion of kitchen garden and household consumption of its production; initiation and scale-up of child pan concept whereby children aged from 6 to 24 months would be having an adequate meal for their appropriate nutrition; provision of

584 cows to 584 households with severely malnourished children; provision of 1548 small livestock to 1548 households with severely malnourished children; promotion of household production and/or consumption of micronutrient-rich foods; sensitization of pregnant women on the benefit of doing 4 antenatal care (ANC) visits; promotion of hand washing; use of latrines; use of "step and wash" technology ; personal hygiene; use of clean kitchen utensils; use of dish rack; access to potable water; rainwater harvesting; hygiene and sanitation in schools; promotion of family planning; provision of meals in all school going children; provision of a cup of milk twice a week to all school going children-nursery to primary 3; deworming campaigns in nursery and primary schools; hand washing in primary schools; micronutrient supplementation to all nursery and primary school children; identification and dissemination of the best practices in agriculture that enhance food security and nutrition; promotion of dietary diversity including vegetables, fruits and animal source foods to enhance food and nutrition security; promotion of income generating activities to enhance food and nutrition security; promotion of fish farming to improve protein intake; promotion of one rabbit/one child to improve protein intake; promotion of potable drinking water and regular monitoring system. After each daily work period, participants to the elaboration of the plan had to go for relax and entertainment in the town of RUSIZI in western province of Rwanda, and that town is at one of the borders between Rwanda and Democratic Republic of Congo . One time at around 8 pm local time, there was an issue whereby grenades were

thrown in the town of RUSIZI and those grenades exploded. I was in an internet cafe and I had a phone call from one of the participants who told me that one of the grenades exploded near him. He told me that he was with others, fortunately no one of them had an injury and they had to run away. I told them, through the one who phoned me, to remain calm and to go to their respective hotels so that they could avoid any risks from any other grenade explosions. Those grenades were thrown and exploded by people who may have come from the neighboring country of Democratic Republic of Congo. The following day, I had a meeting with all participants on their security and before starting the nutrition plan work. I had to confirm that all were present and safe, after having confirmed it, I had to advise them that they would reduce their movements in the night. The objective was to work on the plan and to go back to our workplace without any unfortunate events. However, at the end of our nutrition plan, I had to take all participants to a trip to an island located in lake Kivu. There were some boats that had to take all participants to the nice island where local people were waiting for us. Those boats had engines and every participant had a life jacket in the boats. We could safely reach the island and as we were many, the boats had to travel on water several times from the mainland to the island and back, doing back-and-forth travel. Local people were welcoming us by local dances and we appreciated how they had shown us happiness at our arrival. It was a party at the end of our plan on malnutrition and there was a hired DJ with music equipment. The DJ allowed us to have nice music and all people who were present started to dance. There were representatives of the hospital, health centers, district, ministry of health and other partners such as UNICEF. All those people were enjoying the party and after some time, we had lunch and followed speeches that were mainly thanking the work done and how things were organized. We had group photos and at the end of the party, at around 8PM, we went back to the mainland from the island. The following day each and every participant had a soft copy of the work done for any corrections and we went back to our different workplaces.

On the other hand, after the final document of the district plan to eliminate malnutrition, it was presented to the board of directors of the hospital. After being approved by the hospital board of directors, the plan on eliminating malnutrition was sent to the district for its approval and finally, it was sent to the ministry of health for final approval. After the final approval step, there was a dissemination meeting of all partners from the community representatives, health center representatives, hospital representatives, district authorities, ministry of health representatives and non-governmental organizations working in the district as well as other organizations such as UNICEF representatives. All participants appreciated the work done and they were committed to implement the plan to eliminate malnutrition in the district according to the schedule. Many other meetings were held at the district level and sensitization on eliminating malnutrition was one of the topics. I remember that I participated in a meeting in one of the sectors of the district and that meeting was organized by one of Christian churches in the district. There were many local people of the sector and a balanced diet was prepared and given to children in terms of population sensitization on the appropriate and available diet that would eliminate malnutrition. I had to take that opportunity and I explained the balanced diet that is comprised of appropriate proportions of carbohydrates, proteins, fats, minerals, vitamins, water for good health and eliminating malnutrition. I told them that as they had prepared the balanced diet from foods found locally, all the needed nutrients were found in the foods and drinks that they had. I gave them some examples of foods that were available locally and drinks that could make a balanced diet such as milk, eggs, beans, sweet potatoes, vegetables, fruits and water to name but a few. People were convinced and they were committed to consume balanced diet for elimination of malnutrition. I could put the nutrition topic on agenda of coordination meeting, which was a meeting between the hospital and the health centers with some representatives from the district, and that meeting was chaired by the director of the hospital. There were monitoring and evaluation of activities in the plan to eliminate malnutrition and health professionals with weaknesses were requested to put more efforts in their implementation. There were achievements at the end of the district plan to eliminate malnutrition and in NYARUGURU district, stunting, or too short for their age, among children under 5 years of age, decreased from 45.5% in 2010 according to Rwanda Demographic Health Survey of 2010 (RDHS 2010) to 42% in 2014 according to Rwanda Demographic Health Survey of 2014-2015 (RDHS 2014-2015). The acute malnutrition in the district, wasting, or too thin for their height, for children under age 5 in the above mentioned district, decreased from 5.8% in 2010 according to RDHS 2010 to 3% in 2014 according to RDHS 2014-2015.

On the other hand, there was a necessity in terms of infrastructure even if an improvement was already there, at MUNINI hospital, after having built a second theatre operating room and laundry. I had an idea of doing advocacy of funding construction of new MUNINI hospital to partners. The Kuwait Fund accepted to consider the request. A delegation from the Kuwait Fund came to Rwanda to see the location of MUNINI and assess the reasons why the funds would be given for the construction of a hospital at that place. Among criteria for getting funded, there was a necessity of new hospital construction and I had shown it. I knew that the delegation from Kuwait Fund would come to MUNINI hospital the following day for final assessment while I was on my way to an official meeting in Kigali. After that meeting at around 7PM, I had to go back to my workplace and prepare a presentation to the guests from Kuwait. At their arrival, I welcomed them and I presented to them that the MUNINI hospital started in 2008 and it was the only hospital in the whole NYARUGURU district of about 300,000 population (Rwanda Population Census, 2012), 1010 square kilometers, 14 sectors and 16 health centers referring to the only one existing hospital. I told them that infrastructure were not appropriate, they were not enough as the MUNINI hospital was working in rehabilitated houses built in 1986 that were belonging to an agricultural project, DANK or agricultural development for NSHILI- KIVU, and lacking intensive care unit, ophthalmology department and so on and so forth with only 65 beds. As the population in the catchment area of the hospital was about 300,000 in 2012, which was meaning that 1 bed was for 300,000/65 equivalent to 4615 people while it took about 1 hour and half to transfer patients from MUNINI hospital to BUTARE University Teaching hospital. I showed them that if the hospital had more beds, transfers would decrease and we would save many lives because some patients died on the way to the university teaching hospital located very far. I told them that some departments of the hospital were located in the nearest health center and those departments were internal medicine, radiography, human resources, accounting, supervision and the store of the hospital. I also mentioned in that presentation that the hospital didn't have enough equipment and it was lacking anesthesia machine, equipment for emergency cases, monitoring machines in the maternity department, resuscitation trolley in pediatrics, enough functional incubators, appropriate autoclave and an appropriate generator. However, I told them that we had achievements despite all challenges, for example based on kangaroo method, we had decreased neonatal death rate from 77/1000 in 2010 to 25/1000 in less than 1 year and to 3/1000 in June 2013. Other achievements that I mentioned in the presentation were how we had decreased maternal deaths from 4 in 2010 to 0 in 2011 due to a good follow-up of our patients, the way we had decreased confirmed malaria cases from 11,983 in 2010 to 2,886 in 2012 due to a sensitization of the population to use insecticide treated nets, how we were buying food, soap and community based health insurance for indigent patients due to 1% monthly salary contribution of the MUNINI hospital staff.

Furthermore, I told the representatives of Kuwait Fund that despite many challenges, we managed to work hard and we had been the best in terms of service delivery nationwide for the year 2011 according to what the prime minister of Rwanda, then, declared in his 2012 meeting with all directors of hospitals. On the other hand, we could have 100% in customer care evaluation done by the ministry of health and it was in March 2013. Representatives of Kuwait Fund were impressed by our achievements despite many challenges at our hospital. One of them asked me if neonatal death rate had not decreased before the kangaroo method, I answered him that it had not decreased because there was no electricity permanently and the kangaroo method helped us to decrease neonatal deaths tremendously. The leader of the delegation said that they would not only finance the construction of a new hospital at MUNINI but also they would buy new ambulances and they could contribute in the construction of asphalted roads towards the new hospital. Initially the offer was three million, six hundred thousand Kuwaiti Dinar (3,600,000KWD) equivalent to about twelve million United States Dollars (US$12,000,000) or about eleven billion Rwandan Francs (11,000,000,000RWF). The offered amount had to be used for buildings, equipment and other expenses. I thanked them for having accepted to offer such important and helpful funds, to the MUNINI hospital, and those funds would allow us to have an appropriate hospital and to save human lives in that part of the world.

I had to find architects and engineers who would design an appropriate hospital and the ones that I had in my mind were those working for MASS Design Group, a world-renowned American company. I had to find some contacts from MASS Design Group and I remember that I met one of its architects at a hotel in Kigali called NOVOTEL, the ex-MERIDIEN hotel. I myself introduced to him, he told me his name and what he was doing in the company and I told him that I had an idea of having an appropriate hospital at MUNINI. I further told him that I had known that MASS Design Group was doing well in terms of design of buildings. I informed him that there was a huge project at MUNNI whereby a new hospital was going to be designed, built and equipped for an amount of 12 million US Dollars equivalent to 11 billion Rwandan Francs. He was very interested in the project and happy about it. He told me that MASS Design Group would be able to do a nice and specific design for the new MUNINI hospital. On the other hand, I did advocacy of the hospital design done by MASS Design Group to the ministry of health, which accepted that the mentioned company would make a design for the new hospital. There have been many meetings on the new MUNINI hospital design and those meetings were between representatives of the ministry of health, the district, the hospital and MASS Design Group. The first meeting was held on December 23, 2014 and it was aiming at reviewing the MUNINI hospital design. On introduction, it was mentioned that the consultancy services for the architectural and technical design for MUNINI district hospital had been offered by MASS DESIGN GROUP consultants Ltd on behalf of the Ministry of Health of Rwanda. The consultant had submitted a detailed technical design and an estimate of the project that was about 12 billion Rwandan Francs. This was found to be highly expensive and consequently not affordable. Therefore, the Ministry of Health had decided to review the design either by scaling down the project or by changing the proposed materials so that an affordable and final design would be produced by the Ministry of Health on a budget of about 6.5 billion Rwandan Francs. It was mentioned that this was the reason why on that date of December 23, 2014 a joint technical team from the Ministry of health (MOH), Rwanda Biomedical Center (RBC) and MUNINI hospital, met to analyze and review the submitted detailed technical design and thereafter find out how to scale down the project and print the final document for the tender to be launched. On the review of the design, there were first of all, some key facts. For example, the budget for the construction works of the project should not exceed 6.5 billion Rwandan Francs all taxes excluded as per Memorandum of Understanding (MOU) signed between the government of Rwanda and Kuwait, the estimated cost of about 12 billion Rwandan Francs, value-added taxes (VAT) included, should inevitably be reduced to meet the budget of 6.5 billion Rwandan Francs VAT excluded and the capacity of the hospital of 300 beds shall not be changed. Secondly, there were some points for methodology used to review the proposal of the consultant. For example, the team had to analyze and compare the cost estimate presented by the consultant and the budget provided by the Ministry of Health. The team had to analyze the signed MOU between the government of Rwanda and Kuwait especially the clause on taxes whereby the project was planned to be all taxes exempted. Furthermore, the team had to analyze the proposed construction materials to be used and their cost. It had to analyze the size of the rooms compared to their occupancies and see if there were no wasted spaces. The team had to analyze the design itself and see if the submitted design covered all necessaries and its complexity. Finally, the team had to compare the proposed rates by the consultant on various items to normal rates on market. On the other hand, the team proposed some remedial solutions and there were some actions that would be considered by the consultant. On general observations and recommendations, the first action to be considered by the consultant was, the project must be taxes exempted and therefore the proposed rates by the consultant should be reviewed by removing taxes. The output was, the cost of the project would decrease from 12 billion Rwandan Francs to 10 billion Rwandan Francs. Another action to be considered by the consultant was, the proposed rates for ceramic tiles were too high and should not be more than 20,000 per square meter and the output was, this would help to reduce the total cost. Another action was, keep the ceiling only where mechanical ventilations shall be installed and the output was, this would reduce the cost of the project generally. The following example was, change the thickness of glasses from 6mm to 4mm and this would reduce the cost of the project generally. Another action was to review the rates used for doors and their accessories because the proposed rates by the consultant were found too high and this would reduce the cost of the project generally. The team recommended to reduce the height of internal and external walls and make maximum of 3.5m instead of 3.8m, which will also reduce the height of the openings and reduce the cost of the project. The team proposed to change the roof, which would be in metallic hollow tubes and corrugated iron sheets BG 28 instead of using reinforced cement concrete (RCC) slab roofs, which would reduce the cost of the project, too. Another recommendation was, the exterior works should be reviewed where only the parking for 20 cars should be paved and the output was, this would reduce the cost of the project generally.

After those general observations and recommendations in the proposed remedial solutions, there was a number two on reviewing the design itself. As there were different blocks with more than one level, in the design, the team started by reviewing block A, level 0. On the latter, the team, first of all, recommended to redesign the physiotherapy block by removing some partition walls to provide an enough ventilated hall with access to the sanitary space. Secondly, to redesign the dental department by changing four consultation rooms into two big consultation rooms where dental chairs could fit and to provide toilets. Thirdly, to move the family planning room to the maternity block. Fourthly, to reduce the Kangaroo mother care and to accommodate the recovery space. On block A, level 1, there should be provided a window at the nursing station. The operating theatre block should be redesigned because general principles of patient, material and staff flows were not respected and the infection control principles were missing. The recovery room was missing and the sterilization process was not respecting the standards for infection control. On Z block, the team mentioned that the proposed post trauma space located at the gynecology, should be linked with the surgery or emergency. On X block, the lab department had to be redesigned by finding the space for biochemistry, tuberculosis (TB) and parasitology within the available space and rooms for sample collection had to be reduced not to more than 2 rooms to give space to other services. The team proposed to have a separate space for TB sample collection and to have an emergency shower in the corridor as well as an emergency exit. On X block, level II, laundry department, the door between the laundry area and ironing had to be cancelled. The sizes of the doors in general had to be decided considering the types and sizes of equipment and machines to be installed inside. On X block, level II, emergency and operating rooms, the team proposed to have a space for dirty materials and a space for clean materials. It proposed to have a central sterilization block. It recommended to put the operating rooms near the recovery room and a rear dirty corridor had to be created to assure the evacuation of dirty materials from the operating rooms for the infection control. On Y block, in pediatrics, in addition to the hospitalization wards, only 4 private rooms had to be kept there and the wing of 10 private rooms had to be cancelled. On Y block, in imaging department, the doors and windows had to be covered by leaded sheets and even the wall had to provide rays isolation properties. The imaging block had to be on the ground floor due to the weight of the X-ray machine to facilitate its installation. Generally, in all wards, the number of toilets had to be matched with the number of users and all toilets had to be naturally ventilated. Furthermore, offices of heads of departments had to be in their concerned departments and not in the administration block. Only the parking of 20 cars had to be paved and the remaining space had to be left green. The oxygen plant and the incinerator block had to be separated and the maintenance workshop to have its place because it was missing. As the study done had to provide modern, adaptable hospital master plans for both hilly and flat terrains, the team mentioned that the delivered documents didn't show two options of those terrains. Thus, it was needed to provide the entire layout of hospitals showing the entire patient floor on both terrains and the proposed typical plans had to be affordable. Finally, the team concluded by mentioning that the review of the MUNINI hospital design had to keep 300 beds, to consider affordable and economic materials and not exceed the available budget.

Another meeting was held on May 7, 2015 and it was for an analysis of the final documents for consultancy services of MUNINI hospital and typical hospital master plans design, for hilly and flat areas on behalf of the ministry of health of Rwanda. In the meeting there were representatives from the ministry of health (MOH), Rwanda Biomedical Center (RBC), MASS Design Group and MUNINI hospital and the team had to analyze the submitted corrected documents. On the background of the project, it was mentioned that according to the terms of references, the consultancy had to submit the following deliverables of a typical plan of hilly and flat terrains: architectural plans (floor plans, elevations, sections and perspectives), structural designs (foundations, columns, beams and slab, roof structure), electrical and mechanical designs, medical equipment plan, external works and tender document. After awarding the tender to MASS Design

Group, it was better to specify the site in order to provide a complete set of documents, from the preliminary report to the tender document and MUNINI Hospital was selected. In contract negotiation, MUNINI hospital was included in addition to what was requested in the tender documents and the deliverables were: one complete set of designs and drawings ready for the construction of MUNINI hospital, two sets of typical designs and drawings for flat and hilly terrains reproduced from MUNINI hospital designs that can be replicated elsewhere in the country, and hard copied and electronic copies. After analysis of all deliverables, the technical team found the following: On MUNINI hospital, there were geotechnical survey, soil infiltration test, costing of works, bill of quantities, technical specifications, environmental impact assessment, structure calculation, architectural plans, civil plans, structural plans, mechanical plans, electrical plans and plumbing plans. On two typical designs for hilly and flat terrains, there were typical plan (schematic layout) for hilly and flat terrains, architectural plans (floor plans, elevations, sections and perspectives), modular typical floor plan (departments separately designed each other), and electrical and mechanical designs. After analyzing all documents, the team found that the consultant submitted the typical plans for hilly and flat areas as well as the detailed architectural and technical plans for MUNINI hospital according to the terms of reference of the contract reference REP 36/S/2011-N/MINISANTE-KFW. Therefore, the final documents were approved.

From July 21 to July 22, 2015, there was a meeting on final validation of master plan and detailed design of MUNINI hospital and typical plans of district hospital. The observations on typical design plans for district hospitals were on architectural drawings based on patient flow. With regard the reception area, the comments were to provide windows for natural ventilation and lighting in medical record store or archive; to provide a work desk inside the archive room and to precise the size of the waiting area according to the demand. With regard public toilets floor plans, the consultant had to make sure that natural ventilation was provided. On maternity block, consultation rooms in maternity had to be the typical consultation rooms in gynecology; the labor room had to be different from the pre-delivery room; the internal configuration of the operating rooms had to be readjusted in order to respect the proper flow of patients, staff and materials and to provide a central sterilization block for the entire hospital, which had to be located near the operating rooms for maternity and general surgery. On neonatal intensive care unit, the consultant had to create a small room, in the designed nursing station, which had to be a changing room for visitors. With regard the laboratory block, the consultant had to provide a private room for gynecology sample collection; a parasitology room had to be included in the design; the consultant had to create a waiting area, for tuberculosis (TB) patients, which had to be separated from other waiting areas of the laboratory and the National Reference Laboratory (NRL) had to provide new norms and standards to the design for reference. On emergency room, the consultant had to provide dirty room to store dirty linens; two isolation rooms including toilets and bathrooms had to be provided. On Imaging, it was needed a changing room in each corner of each X-ray exposure room and an access way from X-ray rooms to processing room had to be created. With regard operating rooms in the surgery, the internal configuration of the operating rooms had to be readjusted in order to respect the proper flow of patients staff and materials. On intensive care unit, it had to contain a technical storage room. Generally, other missing departments such as dentistry, ophthalmology, out-patient department, maintenance workshops, mortuary had to be added. Also small storage rooms for cleaning materials had to be provided in each department. The recommendations for the phasing of MUNINI hospital were, first of all, on mortuary whereby, washing room had to be accessible before the refrigeration's rooms, the space provided had to be reduced for two refrigerators, the height of doors had to be at least 2.40m equivalent to 7.87ft, to allow entrance of refrigerators and the separate entrance for the mortuary had to be provided. On maternity, the delivery rooms had to be adjacent to the operating rooms and the private rooms of maternity had to be interchanged with the operating rooms; cases of fistula had to be separated with other services of maternity and the designed corridor had to be protected with special materials such as aluminums frames and glasses. On the Gender-Based Violence (GBV), the reference had to be the standards of GBV services funded by World Bank and implemented in Rwanda. On mental health, the consultant had to reduce rooms in mental health and provided them to the GBV department. On deliverables, the tender document had to be submitted within 3 weeks. On technical specification of materials, the consultant had to check for opening of doors in critical areas such as in operating room where all air circulations had to be controlled. On structure design, the consultant had to provide dimensions to the foundation plans, which would facilitate the setting out and implementation; the structure plans for the slab had to be provided; the consultant had to provide different types of columns and due to different sizes of columns, the consultant had to provide a table scheduling different sizes and the reinforcement details. On water and water waste system, the consultant had to provide a backup of wastewater treatment plant (WWTP) not only a septic tank and making sure whether water tank was designed. With regard protection, the ministry of health had to provide to the designer, MASS Design Group, the standard for radiation protection. In conclusion, MASS Design Group had to make adjustments to the typical plans and MUNINI hospital design in accordance with the comments made above and to submit the revised documents and the tender document within 3 weeks for the completion of the terms of contract.

Another meeting was held on September 23, 2015 and it was aimed at negotiating on a financial proposal. The meeting was held in a conference room of the ministry of health and there was a joint team of the ministry of health, MUNINI hospital, NYARUGURU district and MASS Design Group representatives. The aim of the meeting was to find out a solution with regard the financial proposal related to the services to be provided by the consultant in phasing the initial design into two phases. According to the meeting held at the ministry of health on May 7, 2015, it was decided to phase the initial design into two phases and the consultant MASS Design Group submitted a financial proposal equivalent to US$93,378. On May 29, 2015, there was another meeting between the representatives of the ministry of health and the representatives of the consultant in order to analyze the submitted financial proposal. During that time it has been noticed that the unit prices used in the amendment financial proposal were similar to those in the initial contract. However, the consultant accepted to reduce some items, which represented a reduction of US$3,930. The consultant also agreed to make a reduction on total remuneration by 20%, which made a reduction of US$17,800. Therefore the negotiated amendment proposal was US$74,850 instead of US$93,378. When the consultant submitted the final financial proposal, he mentioned it was taxes exclusive while the unit prices in the initial proposal were taxes inclusive. Thus, the representatives of the ministry of health rejected that statement of "taxes exclusive." After open discussion, the following were key resolutions from the meeting: On the issue of taxes inclusive or not inclusive in the negotiated financial proposal proposed by Mass Design Group and after discussion and analysis on the initial contract and initial bid document, it was found that the unit prices were with taxes inclusive. Therefore, the consultant agreed that the negotiated financial proposal equivalent to US$74,850 was taxes inclusive. The consultant had to re-submit the new financial proposal of US$74,850 and consider it as taxes inclusive. On the proposal of payments for phasing the initial design into two designs, three installments were proposed and the first payment was 30% of amendment cost, the second one was 40% and the third payment was

30%. The consultant was required to provide the detailed deliverables for each payment installments. However, the payment of the second installment had to be done after the approval of the final document of the phase one. On work plan, the consultant proposed to complete and submit the final document of the first phase within 8 weeks after payment of the last installment of the initial contract. The final document of the phase two to be complete and submitted within 4 weeks after completion of the phase 1. As recommendations, the consultant had to submit the detailed deliverables for each phase and meet the timelines and the ministry of health had to quickly process for the contract amendments and process to the payment of the last installment of the initial contract.

On November 19, 2018 the construction of the New MUNINI hospital was at 25% completion, according to the email message that MASS Design Group sent to me, as progress was moving to the second floor of the first building. The project was planned to be completed in 2020.

CHAPTER XIV

Contribution to the community

On the other hand, I had to contribute to the community at the sector that was near the hospital. As there were many poor people, I had an idea to contribute to the construction of a saving and credit cooperative at the nearest sector. I paid one hundred and twenty thousand Rwandan Francs (120,00Rwf) equivalent to one hundred and forty-one US dollars (US$141), as my contribution, from my salary, to the construction of that financial cooperative. I believed that the saving and credit cooperative would help people to get money and to have businesses that would improve their lifestyle both economically and in terms of welfare. Other staff of the hospital understood the importance of that financial organization and many of them at the hospital level, started to contribute, too. After the construction of the saving and credit cooperative, it was the first financial institution at MUNINI sector and local authorities, business people and the population were very happy. Not only the contribution was provided from the hospital staff to the construction of the financial cooperative, but also, I proposed during a meeting of the management committee to deposit money daily received by the cashier in the saving and credit cooperative of MUNINI instead of keeping that money in the hospital. There were two profits in depositing that money in that financial cooperative: first of all, in terms of security, it was safe to put that money in that cooperative rather than being kept at the hospital level. Secondly, that money helped the cooperative in terms of giving loans to the population in an easy way and without delay. The management committee of the MUNINI hospital accepted the proposal and on January 3, 2015, since 2 years back, the hospital had about US$34,000, equivalent to 29,000,000RWF, of deposit in the MUNINI saving and credit cooperative. That money allowed that financial institution to give loans to the local population. Those who had businesses had an opportunity to extend their activities based on loans provided by the MUNINI saving and credit cooperative. One client of that cooperative said "Actually, the only bank, which was in the NYARUGURU district, was at KIBEHO far from MUNINI and other banks were in other districts such as HUYE and NYAMAGABE. As there was no financial institution at MUNINI, it was very hard to travel to KIBEHO or other districts because of the long distance between MUNINI and those places." All clients of MUNINI saving and credit cooperative said that it was very helpful to them. Three of them could buy cars, which were helping them in their businesses and others could build their own houses. There were other clients of that financial cooperative of MUNINI, who were able to invest in cultivating tea as there was a plan to build a tea factory in that area. The soil is generally acidic, in NYARUGURU district, with a pH between 5 and 5.5 and that soil is favorable to tea agriculture. Tea originated in southwest of China, Sichuan/Yunnan area and recorded in 59BC or Before Christ period. At the beginning, it was used as a medicinal drink before being popularized as a recreational drink during the Chinese Tang dynasty and tea drinking spread to other East Asian countries. Portuguese priests and merchants introduced it to Europe during the 16th century. During the 17th century, drinking tea became fashionable by Britons, who started large-scale production and commercialization of the plant in India. Combined, China and India supplied 62% of the world's tea in 2016. With regard chemical composition, caffeine constitutes about 3% of tea's dry weight and a study found that the caffeine content of 1 g of black tea, ranged from 22 to 28 mg while the caffeine content of 1 g of green tea, ranged from 11 to 20 mg, reflecting a significant difference. The astringency in tea can be attributed to the presence of polyphenols. These are the most abundant compounds in tea leaves, making up to 30-40% of their composition. Tea also contains small amounts of theobromine and theophylline, which are stimulants, and xanthines similar to caffeine. Because of modern environmental pollution, fluoride and aluminium also sometimes occur in tea. Certain types of brick tea made from old leaves and stems have the highest levels. Black and green teas contain no essential nutrients in significant amounts, with the exception of the dietary mineral, manganese at 0.5 mg per cup. Tea leaves contain diverse polyphenols, including flavonoids, epigallocatechins gallate (commonly noted as EGCG) and other catechins. It has been suggested that green and black tea may protect against cancer or other diseases such as obesity or Alzheimer's disease, but the compounds found in green tea have not been conclusively demonstrated to have any effect on human diseases. One human study demonstrated that regular consumption of black tea over four weeks had no beneficial effect in lowering blood cholesterol levels. Many teas are traditionally drunk with milk in cultures where dairy products are consumed. Milk is thought to neutralize remaining tannins and reduce acidity. Tannins are a class of astringent, polyphenolic molecules that bind to and precipitate proteins and various other organic compounds including amino acids and alkaloids. According to NAEB or national agricultural export development board in Rwanda, tea was introduced in Rwanda in 1952 and it is one of Rwandan main cash crops. Among tea produced in Rwanda, there are black tea and green tea. Rwanda tea is planted on hillsides at high altitude (between 1,900 and 2,500m), and on well drained marshes at an altitude between 1,500 and 1,800m. The strategies for tea sector development were tea expansion in terms of area to be increased for example from 15,000 ha in 2012 to 18,000 ha in 2014 and 5 factories had to be completed and operational by 2014. The first tea factory in Rwanda was constructed in 1960 at MULINDI and other factories were constructed after that period. Those factories were constructed at SHAGASHA in 1963, GISAKURA in 1965, PFUNDA in 1965, and CYOHOHA RUKERI (SORWATHE) in 1966 just to name but a few. Other strategies were to support infrastructure related to the factories, which had to be fast tracked and the examples of mentioned infrastructure were roads, energy and water. Among the strategies to increase tea production, there were extending irrigation schemes to tea fields, take measures to prevent soil erosion, encouraging cooperative unions and provision of good quality seedlings. In 2012, new tea fields were established at MUGANZA-KIVU with an acreage of

1089.34 ha, RUTSIRO with 1148.59 ha, KARONGI with 1938.84 and NSHILI KIVU with 509.38 ha just as examples. In 2012, the planned new tea field expansion was in RUTSIRO district with 3,000 ha, NYABIHU district with 6,000 ha, RUBAVU district with 2,000 ha, NYARUGURU district with 3,000 ha, NYAMAGABE district with 2,000 ha, GICUMBI with 1,000 ha and RULINDO DISTRICT with 1,000 ha. In Rwanda, it is produced one of the best quality teas in the world. In 2012, approximately 97.3% was exported in raw form, 60% of Rwanda tea was sold in auctions, 37.3% was sold directly and 2.7% was sold locally. Every week, at the Mombasa auction, the Rwanda tea especially GISOVU BP1 fetched the highest price. The Rwanda tea has gained enormous acceptability of its quality and the factors that contribute to its quality are: Rwanda climate; abundant rainfall of about 2 m per year on average and acidic soils of pH from 4.5 to 5.5. Due to the high-elevated grounds where Rwanda tea grows, its strength, bright color, flavor and consistency in manufacturing, it is renowned all over the world as a superior beverage. Furthermore, nature has endowed Rwanda with the best ecological conditions, making Rwanda tea unique and consistent in quality. There is sufficient and willing labor to produce the tea of quality. Over 72% of the cultivated area in 2012, about 9,071 ha, was situated in the high mountain areas. Rwanda tea was the winner of the tea cupping competition that was held during the African tea convention and exhibition that took place at SAROVA white sands hotel in Mombasa, Kenya from July 20 to July 22, 2011. There are primary and secondary grades of tea and among primary tea grades there is BP1 or Broken Pekoe 1. The value addition in Rwanda is done through tea packaging, green tea processing and tea bags, which are ready for consumption. There is a tea drinking culture in Rwanda and Rwandans have a culture of drinking tea especially in the morning. 99% of tea consumed is black tea and 1% is green tea. Tea is drunk in homes, offices, hotels, and restaurants. In terms of management of tea business in Rwanda, there is a follow-up made on harvesting tea leaves on time in tea cooperatives, there are efforts to reduce fertilizer prices by having tea fertilizers produced in Rwanda, land consolidation for new tea plantations, consideration pruning and replacement of tea fields. In NYARUGURU district, there is acidic soil with a pH from 5 to 5.5, which is favorable to tea agriculture. The rainfall in a year varies between 1,000 and 1,250mm in that district. The annual average temperature is around 20 degree Celsius. Tea agriculture was on 3,797 ha with a productivity of 600kg/ha between 2011 and 2012 in NYARUGURU district. There were 2 tea factories at that time in the district and those factories were at MATA and NSHILI. The first planting season for Unilever tea project was launched in 2017 in NYARUGURU district at MUNINI and KIBEHO sectors. Unilever is a British-Dutch company, which has different products such as food, beverages, cleaning agents and personal care products. It has over 400 brands and in 2017, its revenue was about US$63 billion. Its products are available in around 190 countries. Unilever had signed an agreement with the government of Rwanda to invest US$30 million equivalent to 25.5 billion Rwanda Francs, one year back, in developing two large-scale sites at sectors of

MUNINI and KIBEHO as well as a processing factory. The starting development was in October 2017 with the first planting of 2.5 million tea plants for the planned expansion. It was planned that tea would be planted at around 3,500 ha and around 1,000 jobs created at the two sites. Paul POLMAN, Unilever CEO, said, "When you want to go faster, you go alone but when you want to go far, go together." He further mentioned that the tea project was a demonstration of Unilever's commitment to a long-time sustainable business model that creates value and shared prosperity. He added that the Unilever's investment in Rwanda's tea industry would bring their great tea brands together with smallholder farmers who would benefit from a secure route to markets and sustainable livelihoods for many years to come. In that project, Unilever expropriated 228 households who were resettled by the district of NYARUGURU and Unilever in houses with electricity and water. Those modern houses were in a village, which residents nicknamed "The New Jerusalem." One expropriated resident said he was happy as he had one of the new houses and got a job from poor housing and extreme poverty. In 2017, the NYARUGURU district had 5,337 hectares of tea and producing 3,900 tons a year. On the other hand, due to loans, which were offered by the cooperative at MUNINI, some of its clients had an idea of building houses for rent. They had that idea because there was a plan to build the new hospital of MUNINI, which would have many staff who would need houses to rent. Normally, the hospital had only 2 houses to accommodate the medical director and doctors. Other remaining hospital staff, around 80, were renting houses outside the hospital.

The needed minimum staff would increase with the new hospital and the number of personnel would be at least 115 for the new MUNINI hospital. The number of staff who would rent houses outside the hospital would be more than 110. At least, more 30 houses would be needed outside the hospital as only 80 houses were rented by the 80 hospital staff, then. Those who had the idea of building houses for rent, were right because their houses would have at least hospital staff to rent them especially at the completion of the new hospital building. In supporting the construction of a saving and credit cooperative and requesting the hospital to save money in it, I had in my mind that the fortune was at the bottom of the pyramid.

There is a book that has detailed that concept of the fortune is at the bottom of the pyramid and that book is:"The fortune at the bottom of the pyramid: Eradicating poverty through profits." The book has been written by C.K.PRAHALAD or Coimbatore Krishnarao PRAHALAD and I could find in it how the author described who and what is the bottom of the pyramid. Other concepts detailed in that book are:"Private sector and poverty." whereby it is described the role of the private sector. Another concept found in the book is:"Business and the new social compact." Followed a concept on:"Products and services for the BOP." whereby:"Innovation: Hybrids" is described. In the book, there are details on "Sustainable development: Eco-friendly." Other detailed concepts in the book are:"Education of customers." and "Women are critical for development." just to mention as examples.

On the concept of:"Who and what is the bottom of the pyramid?" The book mentioned:

"There is a lot of discussion on what the Bottom of the Pyramid market is and what constitutes that market. The original definition of the Bottom of the Pyramid was based on a simple premise. The concept was originally introduced to draw attention to the 4-5 billion poor who are unserved or underserved by the large organized private sector, including multinational firms. This group until recently ignored by the private sector, could be a source of much needed vitality and growth." (Page 6).

The idea of the fortune, which is at the Bottom of the Pyramid, is illustrated by the MUNINI hospital, which helped poor people and that hospital had profits from those people. Not only the MUNINI hospital has contributed to the construction and development of the MUNINI saving and credit cooperative, but also the hospital staff contributed 1% of their monthly salary to help indigent patients. Our 1% monthly salary contribution allowed the MUNINI hospital to buy food and soap for the hygiene of those poor patients. When I saw that the population didn't consult at a high number due to lack of insurance, I decided to pay money, which was about US$705 equivalent to 600,000RWF for a community based health insurance of 200 poor people in a meeting of the population. I took that opportunity to sensitize those who were able to pay money for their own insurance and they responded positively. The consequence of having helped the poor people was to have an increase of the number of patients. For example in 2010, we had 7030 patients while in 2011, there were 8012 patients. Thus the income of the hospital increased and in 2010, the average of the amount received was about US$61,150 equivalent to 51,977,500RWF per month while in 2011 that average became US$78,947 equivalent to 67,104,950RWF per month. There was an increase of US$17,797 or 15,127,450RWF on average per month due to our help given to the poor people.

Another interesting concept described in the book is: "Private sector and poverty" whereby details of: "The role of the private sector" are found.

"Until recently, little attention was paid to the role of the private sector in poverty alleviation. The millennium development goals were developed without recognition of the role that the private sector could play. It was later that the social compact with the private sector was formulated by the then Secretary General of the United Nations Mr. Kofi Annan. The pioneering work on the topic was done by a Blue Ribbon commission organized by the United Nations Development Program on private sector and poverty. The report was issued in 2004....The United Nations Development Program is now fully engaged
 with the idea of the private sector's contribution to poverty alleviation." (Page 5).

I agree on that role of the private sector in alleviating poverty. An example is a district in Rwanda called NYAMAGABE. It is in southern province of Rwanda. That district was very poor before 1994. The soil in that district was acidic. What was found in that district was a type of tree used for cooking. Another thing that was found in that district was grass to feed some ruminant mammals like goat and sheep. They didn't have enough cows at that time. They didn't have enough factories and there were no enough hotels. People in that district suffered from hunger and they had poverty. They used to flee from their district and they went to the districts that were richer than NYAMAGABE. There was no private sector that was involved in poverty alleviation and the government at that time was not doing well in terms of solving problems in that district. The reason, of that attitude for that government, was divisionism.

Before 1994 the government of Rwanda, which committed genocide, had a policy based on developing people according to their ethnic groups and regions, to name but a few. Thus, they developed regions that had many Hutu and in particular the north of Rwanda because many people in that government were from the northern part of Rwanda. That government was not as interested in the development of NYAMAGABE district, which had many Tutsi and located in the South of Rwanda, as the government was after 1994. That district was oppressed at a point that in 1994, 50,000 Tutsi were killed by that genocidal government at a place called MURAMBI.

After 1994, the new government of Rwanda has been interested in the NYAMAGABE district. This government started by sensitizing the population, telling people that they should work hard so they could overcome hunger and poverty. The population understood what was said by the leaders and people were committed to work seriously. The government told them to work in cooperatives, which helped them to have some loans aimed at developing their activities for example in agriculture and livestock to name but a few. They developed terraces and used fertilizers to increase their production in agriculture. They started to solve the problem of hunger and the government encouraged them to cultivate tea in some areas and that tea became another source of money for them. The government also started a program of "One cow per family" that was aiming at giving a cow to every poor family starting by the poorest one. This program allowed the population to have cows, which gave people milk and organic fertilizers. Finally, hunger was disappearing completely in that district.

On the other hand, the government sensitized the private sector to contribute in solving problems of the NYAMAGABE district. The government assured them that it would provide all needed infrastructure such as electricity, water, roads, telephones and so on and so forth. It requested the rich people to put their financial efforts to the development of the district and invest in it. A group of rich people decided to put together money and started to invest in some areas for example in the field of tea. There was an increase of the quantity transformed by factories and exported abroad. That field provided money not only to the local population but also to the whole country because even foreign currencies increased at the country level. This alleviated poverty in that district and at the country level. Those rich people also invested in hotels, which provided money to the local population. These hotels allowed the local population to increase their income and the number of people who got jobs increased from those hotels. The private sector also invested in transport, which helped the population to easily move from the district to other districts for their businesses. People from NYAMAGABE district could sell their production outside their district and buy different needed products from other districts without any problems with regard transport. The NYAMAGABE district started to have a good performance among other districts in Rwanda. Normally in Rwanda, mayors on behalf of the whole district go before the president to present what their districts will achieve within one year. After one year, the mayor comes back before the president to present his or her achievements. The NYAMAGABE district, several times, has become the best ranked district in terms of performance achieved in Rwanda. The investments of the private sector contributed to solve the problem of hunger and alleviate poverty. There are no more people fleeing hunger from the NYAMAGABE district nowadays and this example clearly demonstrates the role of private sector in alleviating poverty.

Another concept that I found in the book is: "Business and the new social compact."

"Business leaders who have engaged themselves actively with the Bottom of the Pyramid have started to reexamine the role of business in society. Many CEOs have come to look business with a new lens-the Bottom of the Pyramid's lens....Recently, Bill Gates surprised his colleagues by suggesting that we need to reexamine the role of capitalism. His solution was to move to "creative capitalism." He defined it as there are two great forces of human nature: self-interest and caring for others." (Page 18).

I agree with what is written in the book about how to do business with those poor people. That business can make profits and help poor people. I have an example in Rwanda where it is found a company called MTN Rwanda. This company is among the biggest companies in Rwanda. It is a company that sells cards used in communication. Those cards are called "AIRTIME CARDS." There are several cards including those that cost a lot of money according to financial status of Rwandans. For example there are cards that cost about US$24 or 20,000RWF but there are others that cost less money US$0.6 or 500RWF. Those can be used in communication not only by using a mobile phone but also by connecting to the internet. For example, I had to pay about US$25 or 21,000RWF for internet connection in my phone each month. This helped me because even if I was in a meeting, I could easily receive or send a message by email using my mobile phone. I remember when I was in a meeting, a colleague, who was acting director of a hospital in the northern part of Rwanda, told me an important message on email. He told me that the message was requesting all directors of district hospitals in Rwanda that they had to compete against other interested doctors for the job of district hospital director. I was first of all obliged to confirm that information by asking another director of a hospital located in the eastern part of Rwanda who told me that he had that message in his email box. He sent the message to me and I saw it by using my mobile phone. I could know that the deadline to submit the required documents was the following day and I decided to stop the meeting. I went out from the conference hall and I found all the details of what was needed to be submitted for the position of director of district hospital. To become a candidate, it was required to be at least a medical doctor with an experience of at least 4 years. Other requirements were to have some documents such as a degree and an identity card (ID). Recommendation letters from 2 well known doctors or 2 political leaders were required, too. There was a form to be filled, which was asking the hospital, of choice, where a candidate was choosing to be the director of, the reason of that choice, the curriculum vitae (CV) and training attended. Finally, it was required an application letter to the minister of health. I first of all went to Kigali University Teaching hospital, which was near the hotel where I was attending the meeting. In that hospital, I had many doctors who were my friends. I phoned two of them and I asked them if I could get recommendation letters from them. They accepted to do it for me and I went to meet them. The two doctors gave the two required recommendation letters. I printed the form about the CV and I filled it. After filling the form, I wrote an application letter to the minister of health and I found a copy of my ID card. I remembered that my degree was at home and I went there to find it and all required documents were, therefore, ready. I took them to the ministry of health and I handled the documents to a receptionist. That receptionist received them and showed me a book where I had to sign in. Sometimes later, a message came by email explaining when and where the written exam would be given. I knew it by email while using my mobile phone and I started preparations. Finally, I did the exam and after some days the results were sent by email. Once again I received a message of those results by using my telephone and I was driving from a school located in the hospital catchment area.

I used to go to that school in an outreach program aimed at examining and treating its students. Such a program helped to do early disease detection and treated students as much earlier as possible. Those who were needing further treatment could be transferred even up to the hospital level.

Many students had upper respiratory tract infections and intestinal worms. I used to prescribe an appropriate treatment to those who had upper respiratory tract infections and send those with intestinal worms to a health facility for laboratory test before getting an accurate treatment.

When I had the message of written exam results, I realized that I had succeeded and I knew it due to MTN Rwanda internet connection. After the written exam results, I had another message on interview that I successfully did. on June 20, 2012, I could get the final message of total results, which informed me that I succeeded. By using internet connection from MTN Rwanda, which was in my mobile phone, I knew a lot of important information that I wouldn't have known without it.

On the other hand, even poor people use MTN Rwanda connection in phone calls or sending messages by SMS (Short Message System). MTN Rwanda is the first company of telecommunication, among the existing ones, to have started working in Rwanda and it started in 1998. That company has also helped the Rwandan population in the use of what is called "Rapid SMS." It is known in Rwanda that "Rapid SMS" is a message sent by a community health worker to all levels of health sector requesting help for example an ambulance where needed. A mother may have a problem, during her labor, which can be solved by a c-section. The community health worker sends a "Rapid SMS" and an ambulance goes to bring the mother to the hospital for the caesarean section. This "Rapid SMS," which uses the MTN Rwanda connection, contributed to the achievements in the health sector for the last ten years in Rwanda. For example, maternal mortality rate has decreased from 750/100,000 live births in 2005 according to Rwanda Demographic Health Survey (RDHS) 2005 to 210/100,000 live births in 2015 based on RDHS 2014-2015. Under 5 mortality rate decreased from 152/1000 live births in 2005 according to RDHS 2005 to 50/1000 live births in 2015 according to RDHS 2014-2015. When people are healthy, they can work and with their work, they can produce. With their production, they can buy what they need. For example they can buy airtime cards of a telecommunication company, such as MTN Rwanda, which will have profits from them.

Another concept detailed in the book is: "Products and services for the BOP" whereby another concept: "Innovation: Hybrids" is described.

"More than 70 million Indian children suffer from Iodine Deficiency Disorder (IDD), which can lead to mental retardation. A total of 200 million are at risk. IDD in many parts of Africa is daunting. The primary source of iodine for most Indians is salt, but only 15% of the salt sold in India is iodized. Iodine is added by spraying salt with potassium iodate (KIO3) or potassium iodine (KI) during manufacturing. Salt, to be effective as a carrier of iodine, must retain a minimum of 15 parts per million of iodine. Even iodized salt in India loses its iodine content during the harsh conditions of storage and transportation.... HLL thus decided to try molecular encapsulation. Called K15 (K for potassium, 15ppm), the technology encapsulates iodate particles between inorganic layers protecting iodine from harsh external conditions." (Page 54).

What is said in the book is true. There is an example in Rwanda of a man called Sina Gerard. He lives in northern province of Rwanda, in a district called RULINDO. He was normally a farmer but he had an innovative idea of transforming what he was producing as crops in a way that they could be packed and sold nationwide. He started by transforming fruits into juice, which was packed in bottles with all details showing among other things the expiry date. That juice called "AGASHYA" (which means "THE NEW ONE" in English) is delicious and it is produced from the passion fruit cultivated in his district of RULINDO. Many Rwandans like very much that juice from Sina Gerard's enterprise. I remember when I was with a group of three people from a meeting in a neighboring district of MUSANZE, I stopped my car at Sina Gerard's factory called URWIBUTSO ENTERPRISE. Every one of us bought at least one bottle of the juice because the price of one bottle at the factory was about US$4 or 3,500RWF while in supermarkets in town, that bottle had a cost of about US$5 or 4,500RWF. I personally bought 5 bottles of passion fruit juice from the factory. That juice has been even sold all over the world. A part from that juice, Sina Gerard has transformed a pepper cultivated in his area. He has packed and sold it in different parts of Rwanda. That pepper, from his enterprise URWIBUTSO, is called "AKABANGA" (which means "A SECRET" in English). In different restaurants and supermarkets in Rwanda, we can find that pepper and it is very liked by many Rwandans. He has also started to export that pepper abroad and this brings money for him, the population of his district and the whole country. Sina Gerard has become rich and he has put other products on Rwandan market such as juice of strawberry and wine just to name but a few. Sina Gerard has been awarded many times for his innovations. His work is one of examples that show that innovation is the source of helping people and making profits for enterprises.

Another concept detailed in the book is: "Sustainable development: Eco-friendly."

"Consider the use of water. In the United States, domestic use of water per capita is around 1,932 cubic meters per person per year. In China, it is 461 cubic meters and in India, 640 cubic meters, respectively. There is not enough water available in most parts of the world to support demand. Even if it is available, the quality of water available varies from indifferent to poor. The goal here is not to be alarmists. The BOP will force us to come to terms with the use of resources, in ways that we have not so far. Whether it is in the use of fossil fuels for energy and transportation, water for personal cleanliness, or packaging for safety and aesthetics, ecological sensitivity will become paramount. I believe that more innovative, and sustainable solutions will increasingly emerge from serving the BOP markets than from the developed markets." (Page 57 and Page 58).

I agree with what is mentioned above and, at MUNINI hospital, we have experienced that problem of lacking water. Fortunately, FHI (Family Health International) an American NGO (Non-Governmental Organization) with the ministry of health of Rwanda helped us. With their help, there has been the construction of a big tank of 20 cubic meters and we had clean water in different departments of the hospital. In the past, we could go to a place located at 20 Kilometers far from the hospital, in order to have needed water especially for cleaning.

But with that clean water, it allowed us to decrease not only risk of infection but also expenses.

Another concept described in the book is: "Education of customers."

"More than 40 percent of India is media-dark, so TV-and radio-based messages are inappropriate methods to reach these consumers and educate them on product and service benefits. Not surprisingly, in BOP markets, education is a prerequisite to market development. Consider for example, the incidence of stomach disorders, especially diarrhea among children. More than 2 million children die of this malady every year, a totally preventable cause of death. The cure is as simple as washing one hands with soap before eating.... However, the problem was how to educate people on the need for washing hands with soap and to convey the causality between "clean-looking but unsafe hands" with the stomach disorders...The children often became the most educated in the family on hygiene and, therefore, began educating their parents." (Page 65).

I agree on what it is mentioned above. In Rwanda there is an example of how Rwandans have been educated in terms of having hygiene and fighting against malnutrition. Through community health workers, Rwandans knew the importance of having a good diet and hand washing. This influenced the success experienced in the Rwandan health sector whereby children under age 5 who were underweight decreased from 18% in 2005 according to Rwanda Demographic and Health Survey 2005 (RDHS 2005) to 9%

in 2015 according to Rwanda Demographic and Health Survey 2014-2015 (RDHS 2014-2015).

On the other hand, there is an interesting concept called: "Development as social transformation" where there are details of another concept: "Women are critical for development."

"A well-understood and articulated reality of development is the role of women. Women are central to the entire development process. They are also at the vanguard of social transformation." (Page 134).

In Rwanda, women have been promoted and they have 61% of parliamentary seats since September 4, 2018. The percentage of Rwandan women in parliament is the highest proportion of female in parliament in the world. This is one of factors of positive economic growth of about 7% each year on average in Rwanda, after 1994 Genocide against Tutsi.

In terms of helping the community, I had to propose to the management committee of the hospital that we had to build a house to a survivor, of 1994 genocide against Tutsi, who was in need of it. I told all members of the committee that we would find money for that activity from the indigent account where we put 1% of our monthly salaries. I explained them that helping the community was key for our success as a hospital. Helping people near an institution brings trust from those people to what that institution is doing. Furthermore, poverty decreases among people around the institution and they can be able to request services from it. The management committee of MUNINI hospital accepted to help the survivor of genocide. I had to present the idea to board of directors, which accepted it, too. The survivor was a widow who had one daughter and she lived near the hospital. I went to see her and I told her that the MUNINI hospital was going to build a house, which would include a toilet. She accepted and told me that she would never think that hospital staff could imagine such an amazing idea. The hospital had to find a constructor who was working for it at the hospital level. I told him that we could build a house with a toilet for the survivor and handle it to her during the commemoration of genocide. As we had to give her a cow at that time, I told the constructor to build a place where the cow would be kept. Furthermore, the hospital had to offer her food, help her to open an account in the nearest saving and credit cooperative and put money on her account. The hospital staff, in collaboration with partners in the district, had to work for the construction of the house during a scheduled collective work for the survivor. The total expenses for the help, without taking into account the work done, would be around US$1176 equivalent to 1,000,000RWF.

At the commemoration, a house with electricity and all needed parts such as a toilet and a place to be used for keeping a cow, was ready. There was a cow that was bought in a market of the district, for her. We brought many bags full of different items of food such as rice, beans and Irish potatoes. Moreover, we could buy several liters of cooking oil and a big quantity of soap for the survivor. We gave her about US$118 or 100,000RWF that had to be put in her account, which we had already opened at the nearest saving and credit cooperative. She thanked us so much and told us that she could then sleep in a nice house and have milk from the cow, which would allow her to avoid any risks of malnutrition. There was a journalist who was covering the event from the Rwandan television. I gave him an interview, which he had to take to the television and the interview was published as news, then. In the interview, I told him that we helped the survivor because she was in need of help, which would allow her to live as a human being. I also quoted Martin Luther King JR who said: "Of all the forms of inequality, injustice in health care is the most shocking and inhumane." (Steve Brouwer. (2011). Revolutionary Doctors. Page 215).

Hospital board of directors appreciated the aid given to the survivor and people in the district expressed their gratitude, too. Rwandan television news on the event was highly appreciated by the viewers who thanked MUNINI hospital staff for the charity provided to the survivor of genocide. I was proud of the event and encouraged by the appreciation from different people.

CHAPTER XV

An international journal recognizes
An Excellent Treatment of HIV/AIDS

In Rwanda, at MUNINI there were people living with HIV (PLWHIV) and some of them died while they were on antiretroviral therapy (ART). HIV, human immunodeficiency virus, has signs and symptoms that are in 3 stages. Those stages of HIV are acute HIV infection, clinical latency and AIDS or acquired immunodeficiency syndrome.

In acute HIV infection, many people have flu-like signs and symptoms in about 2 up to 4 weeks after infection of HIV. Those SIGNS and SYMPTOMS in HIV stage I are:

fever; chills; inflammation of the throat; lymph nodes are swollen; fatigue; headache; muscle aches or muscle continuous dull pain or continuous less tense pain; ulcers in the mouth; night sweat; diarrhea; loss of weight and rash or change of the skin's color is possible.

In clinical latency, or the stage II of HIV, there are less signs and symptoms. It is possible to have enlarged lymph nodes, in many parts of the body, that are not painful. This stage can last from ten (10) to fifteen (15) years.

AIDS or acquired immunodeficiency syndrome is the stage III of HIV. There is AIDS after some years following HIV infection. Depending on the individual living with HIV, AIDS can happen after 10 years following HIV infection, less or more than 10 years.

SIGNS and SYMPTOMS of AIDS are:

recurrent fever; chills; night sweats, which are profuse or abundant; rapid weight loss; extreme fatigue; diarrhea for more than a week; prolonged swollen lymph nodes on the neck, in the armpits and groin; unexplained lesions on the tongue, mouth, genitals and anus; inflammation of the esophagus; recurrent infection of the respiratory tract; pulmonary tuberculosis; pneumonia; retinitis; tumors for example sarcoma of Kaposi, Burkitt's lymphoma, cervical cancer; depression; memory loss; encephalitis and meningitis.

Investigations of HIV are HIV tests, CD4 tests, viral load tests, kidney function tests, liver function tests, pancreas function tests and tests based on opportunistic infections for example chest X-ray in case of pulmonary tuberculosis or pneumonia. Other opportunistic infection related investigations are full blood count, laboratory stool analysis test, blood culture, lumbar puncture or taking cerebrospinal fluid (CSF) from the lower part of the back by using a hollow needle and laboratory analysis tests of CSF, ophthalmoscopy or an eye exam by an ophthalmoscope and biopsy for a tumor.

The antiretroviral therapy (ART) is the treatment of HIV and it inhibits or slows the increase of the virus and the progression of the disease in the body. Options of ART are a combination of three (3) antiretroviral drugs: one (1) non-nucleoside reverse transcriptase inhibitor (NNRTI) and two (2) nucleoside reverse transcriptase inhibitor (NRTI).

NNRTI, in a non competitive way, blocks the reverse transcriptase. Examples of NNRTI are efavirenz (EFV) and nevirapine (NVP). NRTI blocks the reverse transcriptase competitively. Examples of NRTI are tenofovir (TDF), lamivudine (3TC), zidovudine (AZT) and emtricitabine (FTC). An example of a combination of 3 antiretroviral drugs as the first line treatment is tenofovir, lamivudine and efavirenz (TDF, 3TC and EFV). A NNRTI can be replaced by a protease inhibitor when there is contraindication of such a NNRTI. For example in the first quarter of pregnancy, the pregnant woman has kaletra instead of efavirenz. The protease inhibitor (PI) inhibits the enzyme called protease. An example of PI is kaletra or lopinavir/ritonavir (LPV,r). Therefore, the first line treatment can be tenofovir, lamivudine and kaletra (TDF, 3TC and LPV,r).

When there is a failure of the first line treatment, then the second line treatment is administered. An example of the second line treatment is: zidovudine, lamivudine and kaletra (AZT, 3TC and LPV,r).

The third line treatment is provided when the second line treatment fails. An example of the third line treatment is: tenofovir, lamivudine, raltegravir, etravirine, darunavir and ritonavir (TDF, 3TC, RAL, ETV, DRV, r).

Furthermore, opportunistic infections have to be treated properly. Examples of opportunistic infections are pulmonary tuberculosis, pneumonia and meningitis.

I remember that four (4) people died in 2011 due to HIV-related diseases. I had a dream of saving human lives through a study that I had to publish in an international journal. The study that I had in mind was on giving cow milk to those people living with HIV. At the end of the study, there was efficacy of cow milk in increasing CD4 for PLWHIV.

I have an example of Nsabimana Emmanuel who was 29 years old. His level of education was primary five. He was a farmer and he was married. He lived at MUNINI sector, the NYARUGURU district in Rwanda. He was HIV positive and he started antiretroviral therapy on May 10, 2010. At the beginning of the study, he had 400 CD4/mm^3 and viral load below 20 RNA copies per ml. He has consumed one liter of cow milk per day for three months, from August 9, 2012 to November 14, 2012. At the end of the study, he had 587 CD4/mm^3 or an increase of 187 CD4/mm^3 in only 3 months. His viral load was below 20 RNA copies per ml at the end of the research.

Furthermore, there were zero (0) deaths of people living with HIV in 2012, the year when the study was done.

In 2013, I had an advanced training of leadership, management and governance, which was provided by Yale university. I told to a professor who was then leading the school of public health in the mentioned university that I would like to publish a study in an international journal. I further told her that the study was on efficacy of a product in the treatment of HIV. She advised me to publish my study in international journal of innovative research and development (IJIRD). I thanked her and I tried to find details of the journal on internet. I found that IJIRD was the right scientific and international study to publish my study in. When I had a meeting, which allowed me to leave my workplace for some days, I was decided to write the article to be published during break time. In fact at my workplace,

I was very busy and focused on the development of my institution of employment. It was very hard for me to work on the publication at that time while I had a lot of work to do at the place of employment. When I completed the article for publication, I wrote to the journal, which responded me positively. I asked whether I could publish my study on efficacy of cow milk in increasing CD4 for People living with HIV in IJIRD. I further asked what were the requirements. The journal responded that I had to pay some amount of American dollars and send my article. As I had a dream of publishing my study in an international and scientific journal, I paid the amount of money and sent the article. After the meeting, I had to go back to my workplace. I knew that sometimes a scientific journal could receive, review an article and refuse to publish it. Otherwise, it was possible that the scientific and international journal could send back the article for corrections.

I would never forget the day when I was with staff in the morning meeting at my place of employment and I received a positive message from the journal. It was the first message from international journal of innovative research and development on my study. In the message, the journal confirmed what I had written in the article and no corrections were needed. I was very happy as my dream became true and I told it to the staff who congratulated me. With the recognition of the journal on my study, I knew that cow milk was an excellent treatment of HIV/AIDS. I had an idea of writing a book to inform the world about such an excellent treatment of HIV/AIDS. That is why I wrote this book.

www.ingramcontent.com/pod-product-compliance
Lightning Source LLC
Chambersburg PA
CBHW030622220526
45463CB00004B/1375